Food Sensitivity Testing

The Principles of Bioresonance and Biofeedback Therapy

Author: Julie Langton Smith MSc

Published by New Generation Publishing in 2018

Copyright © Julie Langton Smith MSc 2018

First Edition

The author asserts the moral right under the Copyright, Designs and Patents Act 1988 to be identified as the author of this work.

All Rights reserved. No part of this publication may be reproduced, stored in a retrieval system or transmitted, in any form or by any means without the prior consent of the author, nor be otherwise circulated in any form of binding or cover other than that which it is published and without a similar condition being imposed on the subsequent purchaser.

Although the author and publisher have made every effort to ensure that the information in this book was correct at press time, the author and publisher do not assume and hereby disclaim any liability to any party for any loss, damage, or disruption caused by errors or omissions, whether such errors or omissions result from negligence, accident, or any other cause.

This book is not intended as a substitute for the medical advice of physicians. The reader should regularly consult a physician in matters relating to his/her health and particularly with respect to any symptoms that may require diagnosis or medical attention.

www.newgeneration-publishing.com

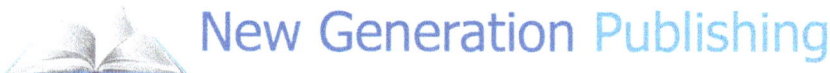

Acknowledgements

Nutritional collaboration from Emma Sewell
Technical Information by Harald Rauer MSc
Charts Supplied courtesy of Bruce Copen Laboratories

Introduction

Food sensitivities, intolerances and allergies have become more common recently and the surge in symptoms such as IBS, fatigue, skin conditions, depression and other health issues have been linked to certain types of foods. Foods such as wheat, gluten, dairy and lactose are among the most common of these foods for people to have tested but obscure foods such as certain spices, herbs, fish, meat, fruit, vegetables and alcohol are also very much involved in some people's health symptoms.

In conventional medical testing, skin-prick testing or elimination of certain foods is used to test for food sensitivities/intolerance/allergies. It is not easy to assess food issues in this way and no medical test is 100% guaranteed to be accurate. It can also be invasive because of blood testing and doesn't always give the patient an answer to their health issues.

Complementary and Alternative Medicine, generally known as CAM, has become increasingly popular in recent years. This book intends to explore in more detail why people are motivated to use a natural approach to their health and in particular the use of biofeedback and bioresonance therapy for food sensitivity testing.

The therapy involves assessing and identifying foods using a hair sample and a digital feedback device, known as biofeedback and bioresonance. This is a complementary and alternative medical approach to helping with health symptoms, particularly with food sensitivities. This book is a guide to help both the practitioner and the general public to understand more about how the therapy works, to experience and obtain best practice for their patients/clients.

Firstly, we explore why complementary medicine has become popular, to give some context to the therapy, and why a practitioner would want to include this treatment into their practice as a standalone therapy, or indeed to become a specialised food sensitivity practitioner.

List of Contents

Chapter 1: The Resurgence and Popularity in Complementary and Alternative Medicine (CAM) and the Importance of recognised qualifications 1

Chapter 2: Biofeedback and Bioresonance Therapy – A New Era of Medicine 6

Chapter 3: Energy Medicine, What is it? 10

Chapter 4: The Theory of Bioresonance and Biofeedback 15

Chapter 5: Technical Information on the Principles of Bioresonance 16

Chapter 6: Some of the Biofeedback and Bioresonance Devices Available 28

Chapter 7: Practical Work 32

Chapter 8: Health Conditions often associated with Food Sensitivities – Understanding the difference between Food Sensitivities, Intolerances and Allergies 44

Chapter 9: Nutrition 56

Chapter 10: Operating Biofeedback and Bioresonance Device 73

Chapter 11: Common Food Sensitivity and Intolerance Tests including information on how to correlate the results – Case Studies 76

Chapter 12: Creating a template letter to send results to a patient/client 116

Chapter 13: Testimonials and Feedback 132

Chapter 14: How to Become a Successful Practitioner 140

Chapter 15 Conclusion: 145

About the Author 150

Acknowledgements and Contributions 152

References: 154

Chapter 1

The Resurgence and Popularity in Complementary and Alternative Medicine (CAM) and the Importance of recognised qualifications

It is interesting and relevant to note that complementary medicine has been on a huge increase over the last twenty years. It is also important to acknowledge this for any would-be or existing CAM practitioner as the statistics are beginning to support the popularity of these natural therapies with the general public. As CAM therapies become more popular, it is vital for any CAM practitioner to be fully trained and qualified. Therapies need a recognised stamp of approval, which is accredited by an awarding body and that this is vetted by the appropriate government education agency. As practitioners become more qualified and offer a standard of practice that both the public and the medical authorities recognise as a quality mark, they will be able to work with confidence and credibility.

The growth of CAM therapies over the last century to present day, a historical overview to demonstrate how health, wellbeing and modern medicine is evolving in the 21st century.

Increasing numbers of people are opting for CAM (Halligan & Aylward, 2006). Many illnesses remain a mystery for both patient and physician. Yet, according to Rothstein, 1995, there is so much evidence that conventional medical healthcare treatment has never been so good. For example, in the USA, one in six infants died in 1900 as opposed to one in one hundred and nine in 1991.

Further evidence in support of this is stated in the following House of Commons report in 1999, that in the UK, there have been significant changes to health improvement over the last hundred years with many advances in medicines and surgical procedures to keep us alive and well – to prolong life. According to this report, 63% of people died before the age of sixty between 1911 and 1915 and only 12% died at the same age in 1999.

Despite these statistics, it would appear that there is a strong resurgence in the use of CAM. Studies in Europe, Australia and the USA have shown that therapies and treatment in CAM is widespread.

A case study into the ethics of complementary therapy research recruitment published in 2009 by the *British Journal of General Practice*, found that in the Western industrialised world, over the last twenty-five years, about 83% of cancer patients have used CAM in conjunction with conventional medicine and about 40% consulted with their own doctor and used both types of modalities to manage their own healthcare in cancer treatment.

The numbers of people seeking CAM therapies has leapt in recent years:

"By 1998, 47.3% of Americans were estimated to have visited a CAM practitioner. Annual visits to these practitioners rose from 427 million in 1990 to 629 million in 1997, indicating a sharp rise in usage of CAM, which has been found to exist in many European nations as well. In France, the use of homeopathy rose from 16% of the population in 1982 to 29% in 1987, and to 36% in 1992. In the United Kingdom, surveys indicate that between 1986 and 1991 alone, the proportion of the British population using CAM increased by 70%. One study showed that nearly 48% of the population in the UK has used some form of CAM, and over 10% have consulted a CAM practitioner in the last year. In addition to the sharp rise in visits to CAM practitioners, the amount of money spent on complementary therapies and medicines annually is increasing considerably." – (Chua & Furnham 2008, p.247–253)

The NHS is also beginning to take CAM seriously:

"In England, with the publication of new National estimates of patient access to CAM via National Health Service (NHS) primary care, there is evidence to show increasing availability of CAM in an NHS setting. However, the term 'CAM' covers a wide-range of therapies and over the counter remedies purchased for lifestyle, as well as for health reasons, and despite the reported changes in patient access via primary care, most CAM-based activity (an estimated 90% in 1998) takes place outside the NHS." – (Thomas & Coleman 2004, p.152–157)

Health experts are confident that the future is looking hopeful for complementary medicine. "Emerging evidence is proving that some alternative therapies are effective in restoring people back to health. It looks like complementary medicine is finally getting the big vote of confidence," said Dr Peter Fisher, clinical director at the Royal London Homoeopathic Hospital. The Department of Health agrees complementary medicine has a part to play in the NHS.
(http://www.dailymail.co.uk/health/article-55405/Why-alternative-treatment-NHS.html#axzz2Kh8Q1amo)

Even with healthcare and mortality rates improving over the last hundred years using conventional methods and medical advancements, it would appear that CAM therapies are on the increase. It is therefore interesting to find out why people are choosing to opt for complementary therapies.

Investigating some of the motivating factors in using CAM therapies

This section includes research by scientists and authors who have investigated complementary medicine in detail and have written about their findings. This work has been referenced individually. This includes qualitative and quantitative studies and provides a foundation for the practitioner to build their own practice and have a sense of offering a complementary medical approach to health and wellbeing that is becoming more popular. It is with this knowledge that CAM therapies may well be a part of everyday work within the health and care sector.

Here you will find a number of interesting articles and quotes that may inspire the reader to investigate further or even carry out their own research. This is encouraged, as CAM therapies are not easy to validate in a clinical environment and this is why anecdotal evidence is available in the form of qualitative studies where the patients have been interviewed about their experiences with CAM.

Why Choose CAM?

The motivations for the resurgence in the use of CAM therapies are that increasing numbers of people opting for CAM are looking for a more 'holistic approach' to their health:

"Currently, the UK is experiencing an epidemic of common health problems among people in receipt of state incapacity benefits and those who consult their general practitioners. Most do not demonstrate a recognisable pathological or organic basis which would account for the subjective complaints they report. As a result, the causes of many illnesses remain a mystery for both patient and physician, with the result that increasing numbers of people are opting for alternative or complementary medicines." – (Halligan and Aylward, 2006)

It would therefore seem that this mind/body link, a 'holistic' or 'integral' approach to ailments may warrant further investigation. There is evidence that this new approach to health is being taken seriously. Dr Goswami, a leading quantum physicist writes: *"At the heart of all illness and healing is consciousness... there is a whole new way of approaching medicine with a greater likelihood of healing called 'Integral Medicine'. This is a new medicine approach and may provide a paradigm shift in medicine."* – (Goswami, 2004)

"We should consider health as having three 'realms': structural, biochemical and psychological." – (Peters, 2005, p.14)

Professor Peters explains that as well as conditions linked to our modern lifestyle, including heart disease, hypertension, and cancer, we have many modern ailments such as depression, phobias, eating disorders, addictions, and compulsions. In other words, we have illnesses that reflect the state of our minds as well as our bodies. – (Peters, 2005)

Research in the Netherlands demonstrates the relevance of a 'holistic approach' to healthcare in their report conducted in the Netherlands in 2010 and published in a paper by Heiligers, de Groot, Koster and van Dulmen (2010). It states as follows:

"In CM, general complaints – as coded in ICPC – appeared to be more often diagnosed especially fatigue, allergic reactions and infections, next to psychological problems and problems with the nervous system. The relatively high prevalence of fatigue may be related to the earlier reported patient's need for seeking CM on specific problems or for a second opinion because fatigue is a complex condition, which may profit from a holistic approach." – (CM= complementary medicine)

As part of investigating the 'holistic' approaches to healthcare, there appears to be a link with a spiritual dimension as another motivating factor for choosing a CAM therapy (Barlow and Lewith 2009). They explain the word 'spiritual' is not meant to refer to any specific religious belief system but is meant in the sense of a more deep and meaningful approach to health that may help to promote a more relaxing state, helping with pain relief, depression and anxiety, encouraging sleep and creating a feeling of inner peace and therefore achieving a sense of wellbeing. This 'whole' approach to health seems to be further argued by Chuan and Furnham, 2008, in that complementary and alternative medicine provides a model concerning health issues that involve a combination of mind and body balance. They report that participants in their study believed that there is a psychological connection to wellbeing and strongly suggests a 'holistic' approach to healthcare.

Other motivating factors for choosing a CAM therapy may be that the amount of time spent with a CAM therapist appears to be longer, according to the research project in the Netherlands carried out in 2010. *"They discovered that time spent with a CAM therapist exceeded that of an appointment with a GP by twice as much."* They carried out a research study where a large number of people consulted forty CAM practitioners and were asked what motivated them to choose this route for their healthcare. The main findings in this report were that people wanted to spend more time discussing their health condition and were looking for a more 'holistic approach'.

"Comparisons in visit length revealed that CM physicians spent at least twice as much time with patients compared to mainstream GP." – (Heiligers, de Groot, Koster and van Dulmen, 2010)

Further to research conducted in 2008 by Chua and Furnham, other motivating factors in opting for CAM include patients wishing to be directly involved in the process of healing their bodies. They want to be cured without side effects, they were disappointed with orthodox medicine, there was more available information on the internet, they had been disappointed with previous conventional medical treatments, they had not had a pleasant experience with conventional medicines and that they did not feel that conventional medicine had a long-term answer to treating chronic diseases especially with regard to pain control. They go on to say that CAM use for the treatment of cancer and HIV is extremely high.

Motivating factors also appear to include having a sense of self-empowerment and taking responsibility of personal healthcare and wellbeing, not wanting to take a reductionist approach to health but preferring to view a more 'holistic' and integrated treatment plan
(Hyland, Lewith and Westoby, 2003). Their findings also mentioned the relevance of the fact that participants were not so much dissatisfied with conventional medicine but felt that CAM provided a more congruent and balanced view that reflected their own values of belief and philosophy.

This section has provided a good introduction to CAM therapies in general and now we look at biofeedback and bioresonance therapy in detail and in particular the very popular subject of 'Food Sensitivity Testing'.

Chapter 2

Biofeedback and Bioresonance Therapy – A New Era of Medicine

What is it?

In simple terms, biofeedback and bioresonance therapy both use 'energy' as the basis of the treatment. They use a sample of hair which is placed into a device; this performs a type of scan that is thought to identify all sorts of health issues that then produces a set of computerised results. We will be looking into this in greater detail as we work through this book.

Any Evidence that it works?
Research has been carried out as a qualitative research project using a blind study involving ten participants at the University of Northampton in 2009. This study did conclude that all the participants had benefitted from this therapy; most had agreed that it was able to assess accurately health symptoms that were later picked up by their GP. None of them felt that it was important to understand how it worked but were pleased that it did. More information is available on these results by request. Over the past twenty years approximately 50,000 food tests have been carried out in the clinic using this method of testing with very good results, in some cases changing the lives of those patients/clients looking for help with health symptoms.

Now let's explore and explain what biofeedback and bioresonance therapy involves, its history, how it is perceived to work, understanding food sensitivities and nutrition in today's world.

History and Early Pioneers

Over the years there have been various terms used to describe this therapy. Radionics was the original name but as the therapy has evolved, developed and become more understood, other terms such as bio energetic medicine, vibrational medicine, electromagnetic medicine, electro-crystal healing, bio-magnetic therapy, bioresonance and holographic imaging and more recently, biofeedback.

Going back to its origins we explore 'radionics'.

'Radionics' derives from the two words – radiation and electronics. This is translated to mean, 'measuring radiation electronically'. It is based on the idea that all matter emits radiation, measuring specific frequencies according to what or who is being assessed. These frequencies or 'energy' is thought to be based on energy similar to that in 'radio waves'. Radionics was the first term used to describe this form of vibrational medicine in the 1900s and was originally created by Albert Abrams (1864–1924). Radionics was used for both healing people, animals, farming and the environment as a way of trying to detect and eradicate pests and toxins.

Albert Abrams (1864–1924)
Abrams claimed that the human nervous system (which is highly electric) reacted to an energy field which carried external information regarding diseases, illnesses and conditions. Different diseases produced different reactions. He investigated these reactions by way of placing wires on the patient and testing by way of using a potentiometer. This was to measure electrical current passing through the body at different rates. After a while he was able to diagnose conditions by using a blood sample even if the patient was miles away. This form of remote testing was thought to be highly unstable by those in the conventional medical field. However, Abrams persisted in his work and forms the basis of 'energy/vibrational medicine' today.

Ruth Drown was a chiropractor (1892–1963) based in Hollywood, USA, who worked with Abrams and followed through with further investigations using 'radionics'. She used a technique that allowed her to treat at a distance, remote healing, anywhere in the world. This was known as radionics broadcasting so it was no longer necessary for a patient to be present. She devised 'rates' for each individual remedy or toxin, pathogen or illness that involved vibrational patterning. These unique rates would be broadcast as a homeopathic remedy although no radio or television was used. It was thought that the vibrational patterning unique to the individual being treated was sent by way of radionics frequencies; these appear to be vibrational energy fields that connect a human being through their own 'morphogenic field' and the individual energies that are around including the earth's magnetic field.

"This is the energy that creates individuals in all phases of life and it is the amount of life force (which is an invisible light passing through the brain, the nervous system and the blood vessels) which animates all these bodies, making one human being healthy and another, through its lack, in a state of dis-ease." – Ruth Drown (ref: Tansley, D. 1977 – Dimensions of Radionics).

Malcolm Rae – Dowsing

(1913–1979) In the beginning Rae worked with the radionics instruments used by both Abrams and Drown. The instruments/devices coded the vibrational fingerprint/identity of any substance in numerical form. Rae was a pioneer in this area of 'magnetic geometry' and converted each substance into its unique numerical formula by dowsing using a pendulum; these movements appeared to be in direct relationship with the earth's magnetic field. Therefore each substance, no matter what it is, has its own unique mathematical equation. He devised a way of doing this by dowsing, using concentric circles and a resolution of each line is at a specific degree. He produced a system of cards, an example of which is below. These were known as Malcolm Rae's rates and based on what is known as magnetic geometry.

These cards build up a picture of the human energy field and any disturbances within it as well as providing a personal remedy to counteract and match any disturbance to produce homeostasis or balance. By dowsing round a circle, Rae discovered that distinct pendulum reactions are obtained at certain angular relations to the earth's magnetic field. These are marked within the circle (see below) as radial lines. The resolution of each line is to one degree of arc. The result is a system of cards, two of which are illustrated below (source: web ref.).

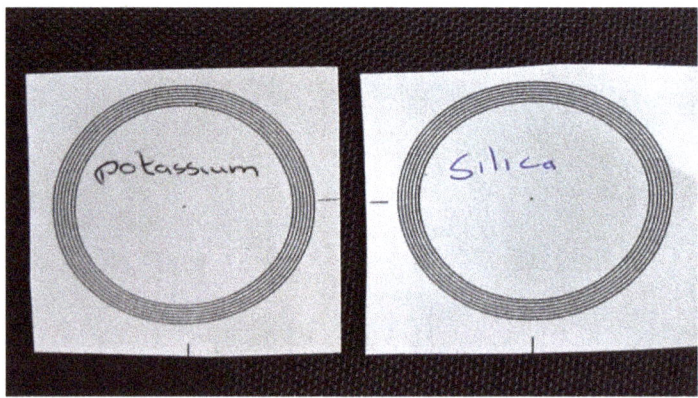

The phenomenon of dowsing is very ancient, possibly dating back to early Neolithic, ancient Egyptian times, but it wasn't until 1240 AD when there are writings that refer to it in more detail. Dowsing was mainly used to divine water with a wooden rod. It is from this that 'medical dowsing' was founded and thus led onto a branch of 'energy medicine' known as 'psionic medicine', which is based on 'informational' inputs that affect the patient's bio field. A diagnostic and therapeutic system developed by Dr George Lawrence in which homeopathic remedies are chosen based on the manner in which a pendulum swings in relationship to a dried spot of a patient's blood. References are available at the end of this manual.

Psionic Medicine

This is another energy medicine therapy based on the understanding that all illness have a cause and that it is this that needs addressing. To find the cause and eliminate the disturbance that has led to the illness is at the root of psionic medicine. Energy thought to be based on psi fields, is understood to involve the body's informational and organisational history. It would involve all aspects of the human being that leads to impact on the physical body such as: the emotional centre, the unconscious mind, the energy centres such as the auric fields and chakras, which collectively is understood as the body's 'morphogenic' field. Finding the cause of any illness is at the forefront of psionic medicine (Reyner, J. Laurence, G. & Upton, C. – 2001 – Psionic Medicine).

Other biofeedback, bioresonance, 'energy' pioneers who have had extensive experience and are knowledgeable in their understanding of healing the whole body with morphogenic field therapy or any other term that means 'energy healing' include: David Tansley, Aubrey Westlake, Dr George Lawrence, J H Reyner, Marjorie de la Warr, Professor Lazlo, Carl Upton, Rupert Sheldrake, Nikola Tesla. Apologies to any other person that has dedicated their life and belief to this area of therapy that been omitted here by the author.

Chapter 3

Energy Medicine, What is it?

Listed here are a number of other complementary medical therapies that are well known and are based on 'energy'.

Acupuncture
This involves the careful insertion of fine needles into specific areas that have been identified by the Chinese to help feed energy through channels to the organs of the body. These areas are known as acupuncture points and the channels are known as meridians.

Ayurveda
Balancing the body system using diet, herbal treatments and yogic breathing, thought to bring a harmony and balance to mind, body and spirit. Based on a Hindu system.

Homeopathy
A therapy that is based on creating substances that mimic the actual disease, taking small doses of these substances is thought to heal the disease creating a 'like for like' healing process.

Naturopathy
A combination of therapies based on natural remedies such as vitamins, minerals, herbs, homeopathy, massage, fasting, water, colon therapy, bioresonance and ozone therapy.

Chiropractic
This therapy is a form of alternative treatment to realign the joints, especially the spine, which is thought to have a direct impact on the health of the nervous system. This is a 'hands on' manipulative style of treatment. This realignment is thought to benefit the body's energy.

Osteopathy
As above, but also involves massage of muscles as well as the manipulation of joints for injuries to help the whole body to repair.

Chinese Medicine
A combination of therapies such as acupuncture, tai chi, herbal medicines, massage that are all based on traditional Chinese techniques.

Tai Chi
A form of exercise that helps the flow of energy through the body, enabling a sense of improvement of mobility and a sense of uplifting of self.

Yoga
Exercise that involves different poses for strength and mobility, involving breathing techniques and a mindful approach to using the body, helping with relaxation.

Electromagnetic Therapy
This therapy is based on balancing the natural electromagnetic fields of the human body with a device that can send a variety of radio waves, electromagnetic waves and other types of electromagnetic energy to either stimulate or sedate the energy fields that have been shown as 'out of balance'.

Reiki
Life force energy, the laying on of hands to help the body to heal through channelling energy to restore health and harmony to the body.

Qigong
Life force energy used in exercise, body movement and posture together with breathing techniques and meditation for health and wellbeing.

Meditation
Thought, mindful concentration to relax and open up the channels of energy within the mind, heart and physical body. A sense of being in a trance or a state of deep relaxation to achieve complete peace.

Hypnosis
This is a state of consciousness that is in between wakefulness and sleep, a trance-like, day dream state, which is thought to allow the unconscious/sub-conscious mind to be open to suggestion. This helps to relieve unwanted thoughts such as anxiety, panic and phobias; also helps with addictive behaviours such as smoking.

Art Therapy
An expressive therapy to help an individual achieve a sense of harmony and balance in mind, body and spirit. Artistic expression may well help to relieve stress through the creative process of using chalks, paints, markers and other materials.

Dance Therapy
The use of movement to relieve feelings of stress, helping with mobility, emotion and thought processes. This therapy provides a therapeutic connection between movement and emotion.

Music Therapy
This therapy is thought to be helpful to all aspects of the physical, emotional and thinking body, producing a sense of uplifting of spirits and creating a sense of harmony in the body. It is also thought that this can help with learning difficulties and mental issues.

Theories surrounding the term 'energy' used in healing

There are many theories describing types of energy involved in the process of 'energy' healing. Here are some ideas from eminent scientists and doctors regarding their understanding of the term 'energy'.

Rupert Sheldrake explains that there are invisible connections such as magnetic fields around the earth and the sun and that these radiate to the earth from distant galaxies through 'electromagnetic fields'. These same types of 'electromagnetic fields' invisibly connect us to other experiences such as television, radio, mobile phones and more recently the internet. He continues to say that radiations are everywhere, whether there is a receiver as listed above or not and explains that this leads on to an assumption that, according to quantum theory, there is a connection between the 'observer and the observed' (Sheldrake 1999). Magnetic waves, radio waves, gravity and those 'invisible' connections are only perceivable due to their effects on other phenomena (Oldfield & Coghill, 1988). They go on to say that this 'non-phenomena' is suspicious in the scientific world, even though it is well known that they exist.

According to Mason (2001), the ability to heal our body seems to be within the vibration of the electromagnetic fields that control the function of cells. If the body has the intelligence in how to heal but fails to do so, he claims that the reason for failure must be due to something in the electromagnetic field. His idea is that BRT has an advantage of being able to delve into these unseen L- Fields and assist in prevention of disease before it manifests into recognisable symptoms.

How it works – understanding energy

The basic theory that underpins biofeedback and bioresonance therapy is that all matter, animate or inanimate, radiates energy. Everything absorbs energy by unique wave fields. These are a combination of geometric, frequency and radiation wave characteristics. A force field that touches other force fields and it is this that enables an experienced practitioner to assess, identify and treat health issues by tuning in to this wave link. Everything has its own wave form and humans have a very complex wave spectrum. Each organ resonates or vibrates at a different frequency. Malcolm Rae and Ruth Drown are just two of the scientists/doctors that created a way of interpreting these waves into algorithms.

As all matter radiates energy and that radiation will differ according to the matter it relates to, this means that each element will have a unique identity, its own unique fingerprint. The radiation or energy levels are converted into a format that is easily understood by a qualified practitioner. A trained, experienced practitioner will be able to identify the results and interpret their meaning based on the levels produced by using the feedback device. Please understand that radiation does not refer to elements such as uranium or other radioactive elements; it is a term used to explain that all matter radiates an energy wave length or field. This will include energy such as electricity and magnetic energy. Resonance means the vibration or communication between all these wave lengths and energy fields.

Quantum Physics

Everything has energy and is made of waves and particles. The word 'quantum' is Greek for 'how much'. Quantum theory is simply for particles to be in two states at the same time, matter and energy. There is no need to go into depth here as quantum physics is a highly debatable area and is very complex. It is enough to say in the field of resonance, where matter and energy are involved, the measurement is translated into a numerical algorithm that then translates into a level which the practitioner can interpret for the patient.

Scalar Waves or Tesla Waves

Nicholas Tesla is responsible for the work in 'scalar waves' or 'zero point energy', which is based on radiant electromagnetic waves which exist in empty space. It is the empty space between the atoms in our bodies and the empty space between the earth and the planets and stars. The waves are thought to contain a source of infinite energy and to be involved in healing the body of disease. There is nothing that can be used to measure these waves; it is more field-like than wave-like and fills the environment imprinting itself on human DNA. It can be generated electronically, magnetically or physically or optically such as in Kirlian photography producing images such as the phantom leaf effect. When the human body is within a scalar field or wave, the person can be either stimulated by the energy or the wave can be used to detect information about the individual's energy pattern by embedding it in its field. Every cell has a crystal structure in its wall which holds an energy charge. The scalar waves are able to be used to both detect and treat an individual when using biofeedback and bioresonance devices.

Chapter 4

The Theory of Bioresonance and Biofeedback

Healthy and unhealthy tissue radiate at different wave lengths or frequencies, which are then picked up by the biofeedback and bioresonance device. This is indicated on the instrument as a 'rate' or ratio, a set of precise numbers that assists in restoring a healthy balance to the body by sending the exact rate of frequencies back to the subject and thereby neutralising any disease patterns. Diseased tissue is thought to be different to that of healthy tissue in that its molecular make up has a different atomic and electronic composition.

This type of therapy is understood by complementary practitioners as a branch of natural medicine that has its base in reading the energy vibrations of an organism. It is thought that each living organism or object radiates and absorbs energy by way of wave lengths or energy fields which indicate certain frequencies as well as radiation-type characteristics. This is thought to be a form of extended force field which is around all matter. See explanation on 'energy'.

It appears that biofeedback and bioresonance therapy provides information regarding the disturbance of energy in the body which is causing disease and then treats it by way of matching its vibrational frequency/energy or rhythm to bring harmony back into the diseased or troubled cell/tissue/organ/organism. Biofeedback/resonance devices send precise energy to people by way of broadcasting healing, tuning in to the subtle energy fields thereby raising the vibrational energy and starting the 'healing process'. There are many different types of biofeedback/resonance devices that help to assess health issues providing a 'vibrational form of therapy for healing'. These instruments, devices or machines may also use some kind of brain/heart energy in tuning in to the unconscious mind, communicating energy between the object and the practitioner. It is therefore important in this therapy to be clear-minded and tuned in to a patient/client before conducting a test.

Chapter 5

Technical Information on the Principles of Bioresonance

Physical outline on Bioresonance
        by Harald Rauer, MSc

Principle of Resonance

'Resonance' in general is a physical phenomenon. It can be observed in various circumstances and arises as an interference of systems with some kind of periodic movements. To understand the principle of resonance we first have to look at the parameters that describe any oscillating system: 'frequency' and 'amplitude'. The 'frequency' is defined as the reciprocal value of the number of full periods per second. Let's assume we have a pendulum that swings from the center to the full left, back to the centre – to the full right and back to the centre again within 1 second. The 'frequency' of such a pendulum could be calculated as:

1 oscillation / 1 Second = 1 Hz

Hz (Hertz) is the physical unit of the frequency, named after the German physicist Heinrich Hertz (1857–1894).

If the pendulum would oscillate with 2 full cycles within a second it would thus be:

2 oscillations / 1 s = 2 Hz

Frequencies in various spectra are around us all the time and in different medias. Sound for example is a periodic movement of the molecules of the air around us. We can hear vibrations, i.e. of the string of a musical instrument in the region of 20 to 20.000 Hz. Another example are our mobile phones. They transmit the signal that carries the internet – data or your voice with an electromagnetic wave with 900 MHz (1MHz = 1 Million Hz) or even 1,8 GHz (1 GHz = Billion Hz). Light is also an electromagnetic wave with a frequency of around 10^{14} Hz (which means 1 with 14 zeros).

Another important parameter is the 'amplitude' or the 'strength' of a signal. If we listen to the radio at low volumes, the sound waves have small 'amplitude', if we turn the volume up, the 'amplitude' of the sound waves becomes larger. The 'amplitude' also refers to the energy that a wave can carry. The higher the amplitude, the more energy can be carried by the particular wave.

Now that we understand two basic terms to describe any oscillating system, we can look at the phenomenon of resonance. Let's imagine, we have a set of tuning forks as illustrated in picture 1. Let's imagine, the tuning fork on the left side is designed to vibrate with 440 Hz. If we strike that tuning fork with a hammer, the air around the fork will start to vibrate, also with 440 Hz. This can cause a second tuning fork nearby, which is also designed to vibrate at 440 Hz to also start swinging. Now, let's imagine a third tuning fork, which is designed to vibrate at a different frequency, i.e. 392 Hz – we will realise that this fork is not going to be triggered to vibrate with the first two forks. This transfer of vibration from one system to another is called 'resonance', but it only occurs, if both systems are able to oscillate with the same frequency (or multiples thereof, as 880 Hz, 1.760 Hz, etc.). This particular frequency that triggers both systems is called 'resonance frequency'.

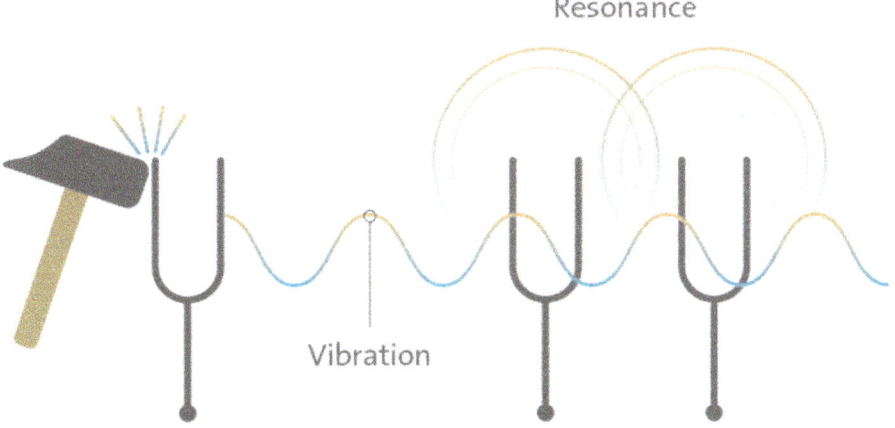

Picture 1: System of tuning forks

Resonance can also have the effect, that the amplitude (the strength) of the original signal gets amplified. Any acoustic instrument, is a good example for that. Let's take a guitar. If you strike a string of your guitar, it will start swinging. Because the body of the (acoustic) guitar is constructed in a way, which it can vibrate with the same frequency as the strings, it 'resonates' with the vibration of the string and will start to vibrate itself so that amplitude of the string vibration is amplified. Picture 2 illustrates that principle, showing the low amplitude of the string vibration on the left side and the amplified vibration of the resonating body.

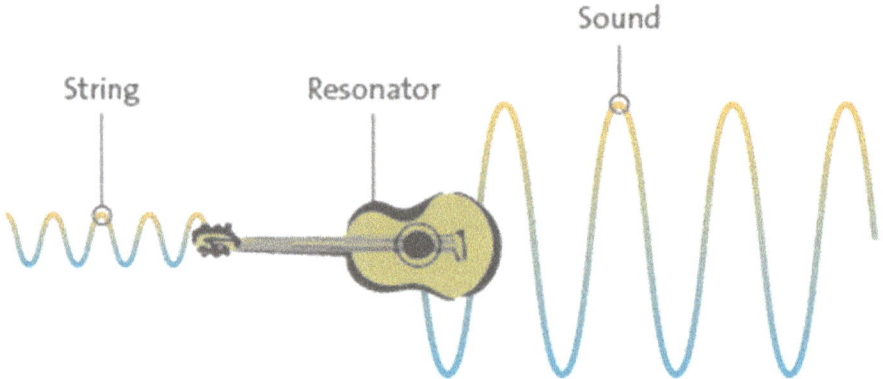

Picture 2: Principle of amplification through resonance

So we can conclude that 'resonance' is a means to amplify any given vibration. By the way, this is something which is not only used in the construction of musical instruments but also in a lot of technical applications like radio and TV, mobile phones. Also quite often engineers struggle with the reverse effect, when they try to dampen resonance as it can have uncomfortable effect on the desired characteristic of a product, i.e. the mechanical resonances of a chassis of a car.

Picture 3 illustrates once more, how the amplitude of a signal can be amplified in a significant way through the principle of resonance, given that the excitation wave and the resonating wave both have the same frequency (the 'resonance frequency' f_R).

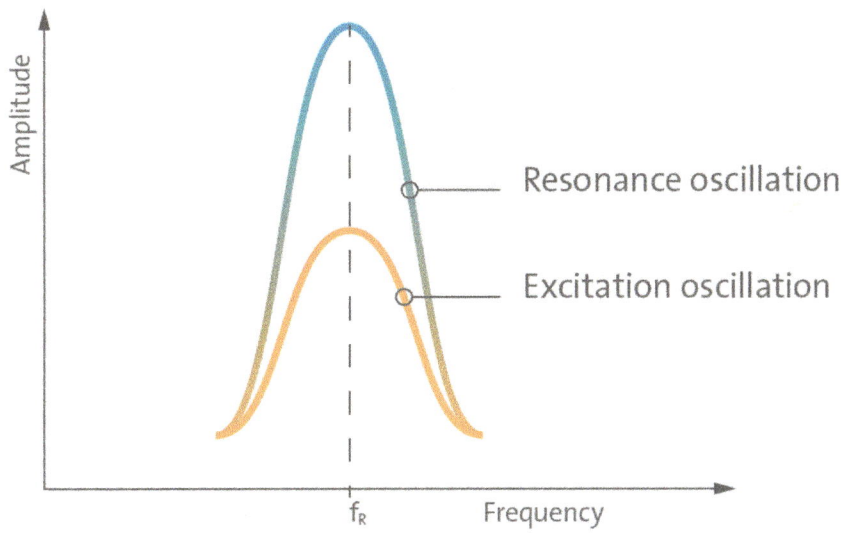

Picture 3: Amplification through resonance

Now, maybe you now already have an idea, what's that got to do with 'bioresonance'. Instead of acoustic waves or electromagnetic waves, we can also use biological signals such as tissue, an environmental poison or a virus and instead of a wooden box as a resonating body we use the cells of the organism.

Therefore we use special devices, called 'bioresonance devices', who have the ability to amplify and detect these signals. As an 'excitation signal' we use test-kits or signatures in computer databases. A small glass – vial with some globules of the homoeopathic remedy 'tuberculinum' or 'arsenicum album' – can i.e. be used as a test kit to identify the tendency to lung diseases or an intoxication of any given patient. Modern devices store the signature of such test kits in a digital way in a database. This can sum up to a number of 60,000 signatures or even more of all areas of medical interest like: organs, diet and nutrition (including vitamins, minerals and amino acids), environmental poisons but also remedies as herbs, homoeopathic remedies, Bach flower essences, teas, etc.

A bioresonance device can make the effect that these very low signals have on our body visible. Therefore we need the patient as such (who puts his hand on hand detectors or handheld electrodes) or a surrogate such as a blood specimen or hair-sample of the patient. Picture 4 shows a typical patient/therapist situation with a modern, computer aided bioresonance device.

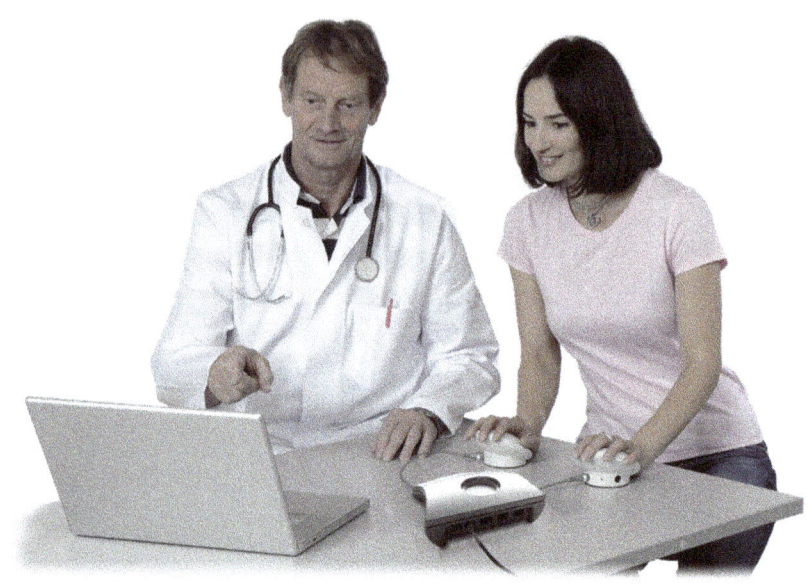

Picture 4: Patient holding her hands on hand applicators in order to run a bioresonance analysis

As illustrated in picture 5, the degree of amplification can also be used as a measure to how much the organism is affected by the micro-organism or toxin, represented by the 'stimulating vibration'. If we use for example the signature of the 'liver' as stimulating vibration and can detect no or just a slight resonance, we know, that everything is OK with the liver. If we use the signature of 'Epstein Barr Virus' and get a strong resonating reaction, we know that the organism is somehow affected by this virus. The degree of resonance can either be measured on a %-scale, reaching from 0-100% or on a +/- scale, having the degree of resonance normalised to a scale of i.e. -10 to 0 to +10 or -50 to 0 to +50 (dependent on the construction of the bioresonance device).

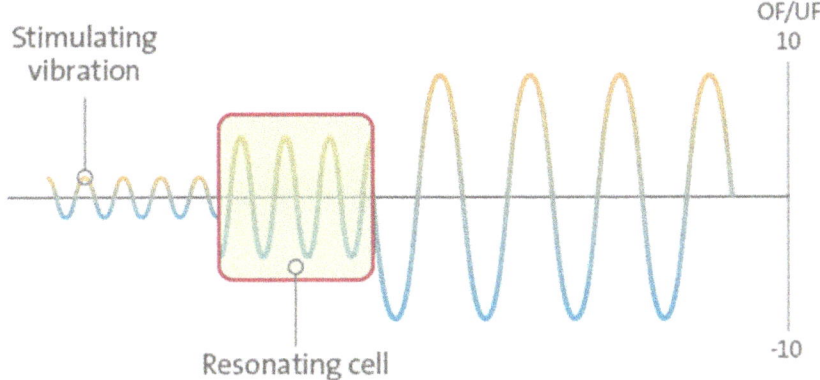

Picture 5: Principle of bioresonance

Cybernetic principles

When bioresonance as a diagnostic means is applied, it reveals the cybernetic principles of our organism. While classical Western medicine follows a rigid and straight 'cause and effect' relation between any disease and its origin, in bioresonance we regard the organism as a complex regulatory system. What is even more important, that it's not a 'closed box', it's an 'open system'. We constantly exchange chemical and biological agents and information with our environment. When we inhale, we take in not only oxygen and a lot of other different gases, but we also might take in micro-organisms (such as bacteria and fungal spores) and toxins and other pollutants. When we exhale, again, we release gas in an altered composition consisting of metabolic byproducts etc. But not only on a biochemical level, also on the cognitive level, we are constantly processing information, sometimes in such an overwhelming amount, that it can create a disease itself (burn-out). Thus our organism constantly thrives towards 'homoeostasis', which refers to the maintenance of a balanced state (equilibrium) of an open dynamic system through internal regulation processes. In that way, a possible definition of disease is the inability of the system to keep a balanced state (homoeostasis). The science behind all kind of regulatory processes is called 'cybernetics'.

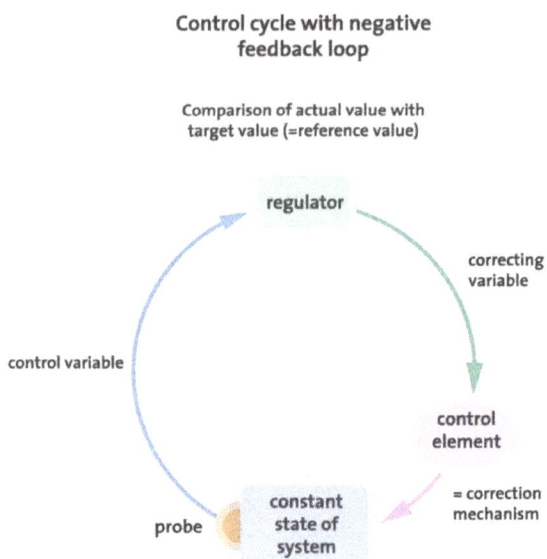

Picture 6: Basic principle of a feedback mechanism

In bioresonance, we apply a 'cybernetic' view on all the physico-chemical processes allowing us an examination of the feedback and control mechanism and the self-organisation of the human body. Picture 6 explains the principle of a cybernetic feedback loop. Let's look for example at our body temperature of approx. 37° C. We can refer to this core temperature as a 'reference' or 'target value'. Now, when we start running, our body starts to heat up through the friction of the muscles, the increased metabolic activity etc. So our body temperature will start to rise. Our body would immediately sense a difference between the 'target value' (of 37° C) and the 'actual value' of i.e. 37.5° C. Through its correction mechanism of 'transpiration' our perspiration glands would produce sweat on our skin leading to evaporative cooling of the organism. This basic feedback loop can be applied to many different processes in our organism.

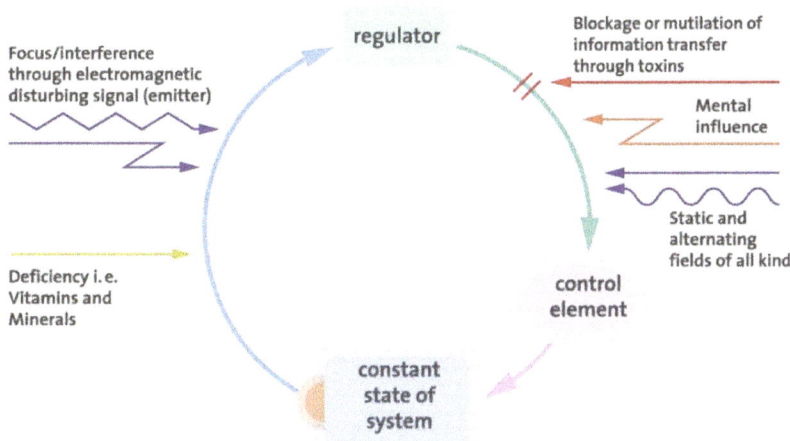

Picture 7: More complex feedback loop in our organism

So as in picture 7 we can take this basic regulatory principle and the basic aim of our organism to keep in an homoeostatic state, on to a more complex level, taking into account all the various influences we are exposed to in every second of our life.

When we run a diagnosis in bioresonance, we observe ONE of several possible patterns on an information level. We use the principle of resonance to determine which parameters (frequency equivalents) we need to bring the system back into a balanced state (homoeostasis). In treatment, we then apply these same parameters to give an isopathic stimulus to the system. Through the resonance principle it's possible to detect not only bacteria, viruses or toxins as in serum diagnostic, we also sense what is affecting the intracellular matrix, the area between the cells, the lymph and the blood (ref. 'basic regulatory system' according to A. Pischinger). Even more, we do sense micro-organisms and toxins not only as biochemical entities, but also as 'energetic signatures' that affect our immune system. This could be compared to the principle of similarity, one of the pillars of homeopathy: substances that cause disease associated symptoms in healthy people also have the ability to cure diseases that produce similar symptoms (similia similibus curantur: similar is cured by similar). This leads to a different perspective on our reality.

The Levels of reality: physical/energetic/information

It is vital to understand, that bioresonance does not apply on the physical level, but on an 'energetic' and 'information' level. This means that we follow the basic assumption, that any biological system does not only exist on a physical (and biochemical) level, but also on an energetic level in terms of a 'subtle energy' or 'vital force' (vis vitae) – in traditional Chinese medicine (TCM) also describes as 'Qi'. TCM has developed a complex system of organic influence in our body, based on the teachings of the five elements (wood, fire, earth, metal, water). This system helps to understand how the organs influence each other on an energetic level. Picture 8 is an example of these 'causal chains', in this example affecting the skin.

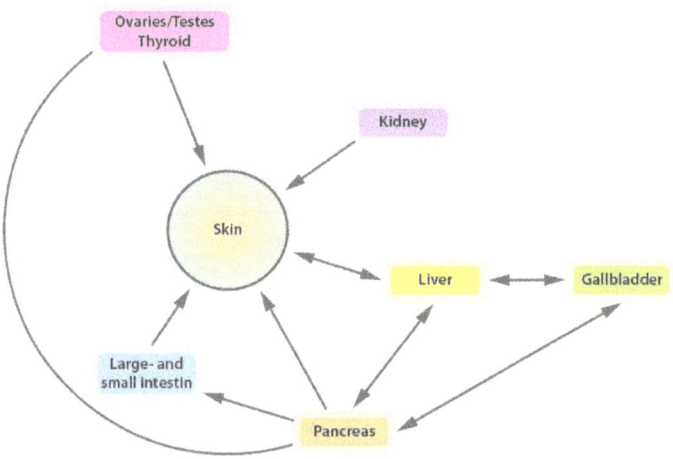

Picture 8: Causal chain of the skin

A bioresonance analysis might reveal that a patient with a chronic skin disease (i.e. eczema) does need treatment of the large intestine or some of the other 'detoxifying' organs as kidney and liver. Apart from these energetic relations and regulation system we have to introduce another layer of reality, which refers to pure 'information'. The idea of this information level is that it contains a blueprint of our organism. The British philosopher and biologist Rupert Sheldrake has used the term "morphogenetic fields" (MGF) to describe these 'control fields' of any living organism. The communicating mechanism between these MGFs and the organism itself, is supposed to be (again) by resonance –

morphogenetic resonance (MGR). Picture 9 illustrates this basic view on our reality as it is approached by bioresonance therapy. This 'information' level is used by several therapies. High potencies of homoeopathic remedies, which contain no molecule of any pharmaceutical substance and still have an action on the organism are supposed to work on this 'information' level. To gain an intrinsic understanding of what 'information' is, let's take this book you hold in your hands as an example. If you would run a chemical analysis of that book you would find cellulose (from the paper), paint, etc. Now, imagine, you would read this book as pdf on your computer or as e-book on your tablet. The physical/chemical analysis would reveal a much more complex composition, of various electronic components, containing silicon, copper, etc. Therefore, even if we can use different carriers (paper, a computer, a tablet), the information that is transferred to your brain through your eyes remains the same. Of course, the carriers have different characteristics, i.e. you need light to read a paper book, whereas your tablet with its self-illuminated screen can also be read at night – on the other hand your paper book won't need to be charged at a mains socket from time to time, but the information remains the same.

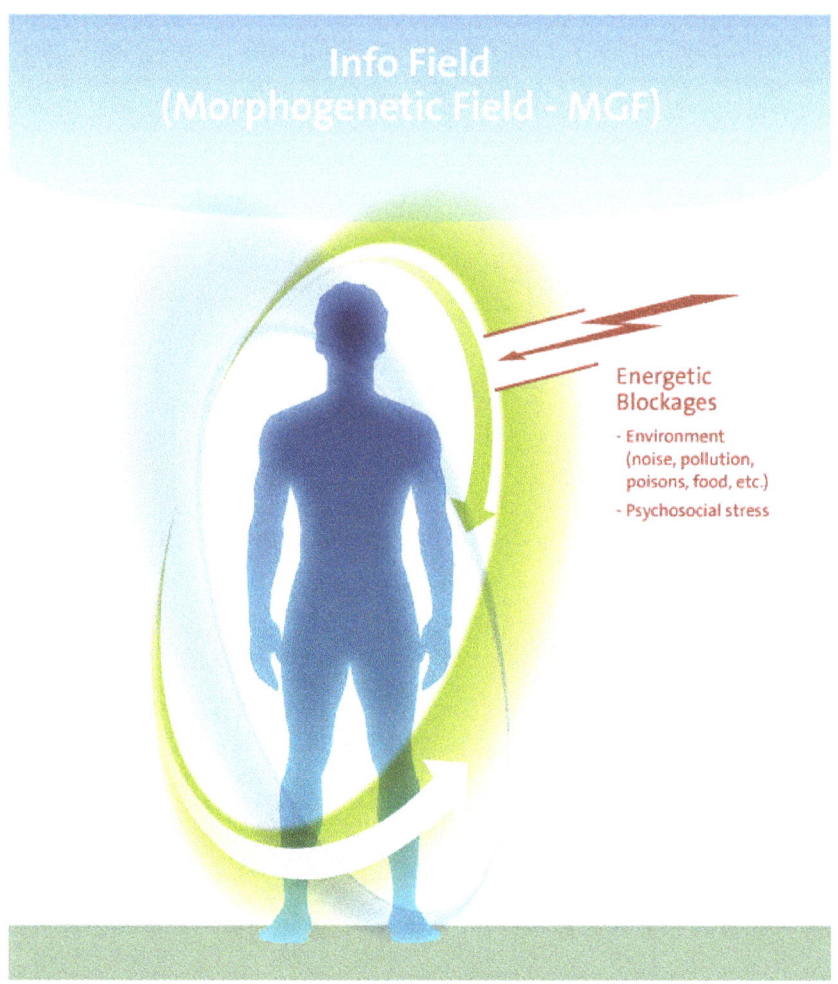

Picture 9: The reality influenced on physical – energetic – and informational level

This brings up another important difference, between 'information' and 'message'. As long as you have learned how to read, you are able to capture the 'information' that these lines contain in terms of different letters and words. But you might not get the 'message' the author wants to get across to you. This could be due to different reasons; maybe you need more information i.e. to understand some terms that the author has used and you're not yet familiar with or not familiar in that particular context. So 'information' is only a means to transfer a 'message' from a 'sender' (in this case the author of this text) to a 'receiver' (you). If the carrier or the particular kind of information cannot be encoded by the receiver, he is not able to get the message. This basic model can also be transferred on your work as a practitioner: you try to find the right information and transfer it to your patient, this information is transferred to the patient/receiver to produce a balanced state (homoeostasis). Bioresonance is a perfect tool for you to gain that in a very time efficient and effective way.

Chapter 6

Some of the Biofeedback and Bioresonance Devices Available

This section looks at some of the different devices available and compares any variations on the use of 'energy', ease of use, science behind them, patient/client friendly, practitioner friendly and the feedback on accuracy.

The Biofeedback and Bioresonance Mechanism and Instrument explained

Multiple Analytical Resonance System MARS lll

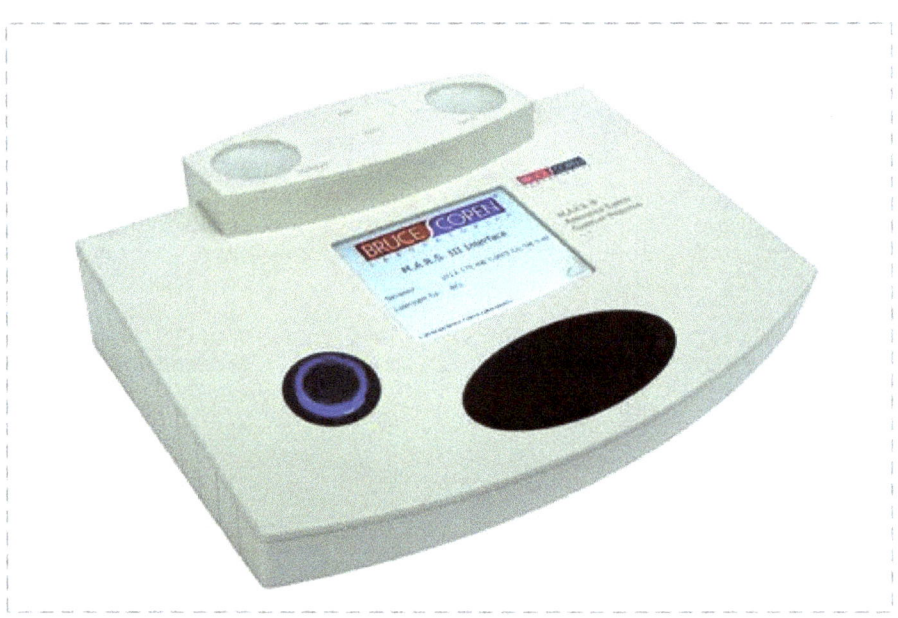

This section describes what the therapy is all about, how the system is thought to work, and how it is used by the therapist.

There are many different types of BRT systems; I am experienced and trained in the use of this particular one called the MARS lll as above.

The following is quoted by Harald Rauer, director of Bruce Copen Labs, (2010), the manufacturer of the 'multiple analytical radionic system:

"The MARS III is a biofeedback device manufactured and has been certified to ISO EN 13485 Annex V standards (2017). The aim of the instrument is, to test a patient on some 60.000 parameters (German database) including organs, micro-organisms, toxins, poisons, food sensitivities and allergens, vitamin deficiencies, diseases, symptoms, Bach flowers and several remedies including homeopathic, gem stones, geopathic stress balancing , electrical sensitivity desensitisation, and acupuncture points. A variety of methods in creating a healing remedy include homeopathic tinctures and tablets, broadcasting rates, electronic card (similar to a credit card with a specific healing barcode imprinted) colour tuning and chakra balancing."

Treatment process

A sample of hair is placed into the biofeedback device and is then scanned into the device together with personal information concerning the patient. An analysis is then carried out which outlines the general energetic balance of the whole body. This is then interpreted by the therapist into a language which can be understood by the patient. There are two types of tests, remote where the patient does not need to be present or face-to-face screening with consultations in a clinic environment. The information is relayed to the patient either in clinic or by telephone followed up with written results. Treatment depends on what the results are. Patients are then advised to carry out recommended treatment, and a follow-up session for monitoring purposes is suggested at approximately three months.

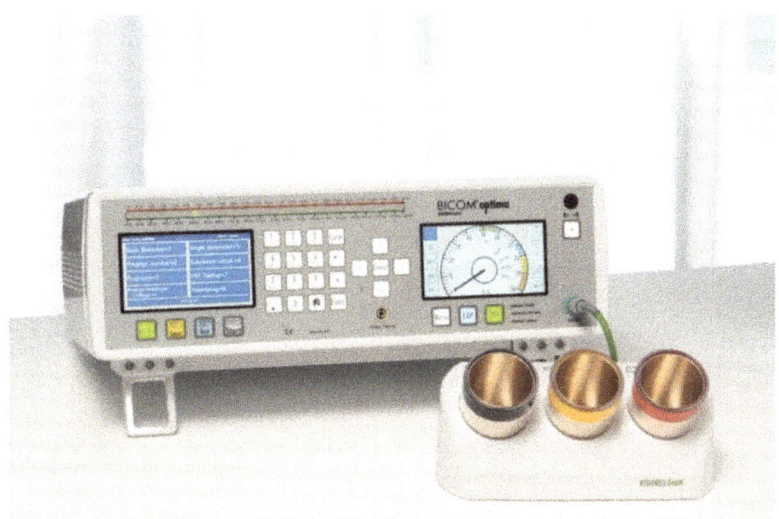

BICOM optima

(Information by courtesy of BICOM – https://bioresonance.com/)

Bicom principles

Living as we do in the communication and information age, it is time we faced up to the fact that the body can only function and regulate itself because communication and thus an exchange of information takes place between the various cells in the body. Research into biophotons is based on the assumption that cells communicate with one another by means of 'flashes of light' (photon radiation). They exchange information over certain frequencies.

Wave-particle duality

Discoveries made in quantum physics have revealed that all particles of matter share the characteristics of both waves and particles. This means that all substances – and therefore all cells, parts of the body, as well as viruses, bacteria, pollen, toxins, etc., – emit electromagnetic waves. Depending upon their nature, all substances have a quite specific typical wavelength or frequency with highly individual characteristics. These are known as a frequency patterns, the Bicom reads these individual electromagnetic signatures.

Bicom Optima

The Bicom is manufactured by Regumed, one of the leading and longest established manufacturers, as of going to print they have over 18,000 practitioners worldwide. It is five devices in one machine which makes it one of the most expensive. It is also not like other devices as it does not rely on a database of stored synthetically-produced frequencies to treat.

Module 1 – Therapy

Unlike other devices it reads the disturbed oscillations produced by pathogens and even the effect on healthy cells. Substances from the patient such as saliva, blood, earwax, hair, stool etc., can be added into the input cup; the information contained is then used for a very individual therapy. Restored frequency patterns and inverted pathogens are returned to the patient. Allergens are also inverted and because of the many thousands of case studies, Regumed are able to legally support the claim of being able to diagnose and treat allergies. With over 1300 pre-set programmes it is very easy for a new therapist to start running programmes.

Module 2 – Substance Complexes

This module is similar to other frequency machines where a stored set therapeutic frequencies can be delivered, but on the Bicom can be administered at the same time as delivering a module 1 therapy.

Module 3 – Dynamic Magnetic Impulse Generator (DMI)
Built-in Schumann generator as used for astronauts, it delivers during a therapy the 7.83hz frequency found in the ionosphere that our cells require to function correctly. This module can be used to bring up or down a person's energetic state.

Module 4 – Electro Acupuncture – EAP
Just like normal acupuncture but without piercing the skin, an audible sound is made when the pen is correctly on a meridian. It is used to measure the energetic value of a meridian and organs and what tested substances are stressing that meridian. Therapeutic frequencies can also be delivered directly to the meridian.

Module 5 – Potentisation
Create your own homeopathic remedies using the typical D3-D1000 scales but in addition to standard substances the therapist can also use information from the patient such as toxins, bacteria, viruses and many other items.

Chapter 7

Practical Work

Hair Sample or Patient Sample, Health Form and Food Lists

In this chapter we start to look at how to correlate the practical work of a therapist/practitioner with working in food sensitivity testing. The symptoms of the patient/client are always at the centre of the testing procedure. The following demonstrates how a practitioner would work with a patient using bioresonance/biofeedback. As there are many devices on the market there will be variations in how a practitioner works, but the following does give a good outline of how the therapy works from a practice point of view.

A Guide to the Process of using a Bioresonance Device

(Please note that there will be different methods of functions with each type of device used.) The following is based on using a Bruce Copen MARS lll device.

Hair Sample or Client/Patient Sample

The hair sample needs to be approximately 1–2cm in length and about 6–10 hairs. It is unnecessary to have big chunks of hair and it is not hygienic to keep the hair. The hair sample must be sent in a clean tissue or envelope, not in tin foil and attach it to the health form. It is important for the practitioner not to contaminate the hair by mixing it with other samples. It is vital for hygiene that once the sample has been used it is thrown away and discarded.

The hair sample works as a 'fingerprint'; once it has been recorded into the biofeedback or bioresonance device, its identity (signature) remains there and can be recalled for future tests. The hair sample is a non-invasive and popular way of working with patients such as children who are concerned about blood tests.

It can be difficult for some patients to understand that the practitioner is not testing the health of the hair and that the therapy depends on the energy, wave-field resonating or vibrating and communicating with the device to provide the results required. It is sometimes easier but not essential to ask for a fresh hair sample to establish a more coherent understanding with the patient about the function of the hair sample. This is left to the practitioner to decide on their own way of working with their patients/clients.

Please note that if head hair is not available for some reason then arm hair, leg hair or finger nails will be acceptable. Again hygiene is extremely important here, always ensure that the sample is wrapped in a clean paper tissue or envelope, plastic is acceptable but no staples or metal.

Here we have the health form that needs to be completed by the patient, which has all the information that correlates with what the device needs in the programme. It is entirely up to each practitioner to design their own health form but it must have the minimum of what the device requires for programming. The more accurate the information being placed into the device, the more accurate the information being received.

Health Form

The practitioner will need to follow the protocol as outlined above to ensure that the patient/client has given them all the information they need to begin testing. See below for a sample health form, which must be completed together with a small sample of the hair.

Health Form

Title		First Name		Last Name	
Full Address					
				Postcode	
Phone				Mobile	
Email					

Date of Birth		Place of Birth including town and country	

Male/Female		Height			Weight	
Occupation				GP Name/Address If known		

Brief medical history (if any)

List of Symptoms (if any)

Specify test purchased: i.e. Wheat. Dairy. Standard Food. Full Health etc:

I agree to my details being kept on the Bioresonance medical scanner database for future testing when necessary. Parents' signature must be given for all patients under the age of 18 years.

Signed ……………………………………………………
Date ……………………………………

REMEMBER TO ENCLOSE A SMALL SAMPLE OF HAIR OR FINGERNAILS
(APPROX. 10 HAIRS 1 CM OR ¼ INCH LENGTH MINIMUM)
Please send the completed form and hair sample to:

Process

The hair sample is placed into the appropriate input space in the device and the automatic scanning procedure begins. This together with the information required regarding the patient/client such as name, address, date of birth and sometimes time of birth, place of birth and a list of the health symptoms, see health form which includes all the relevant information required. This may vary depending on what biofeedback/bioresonance device you have. The health form included here correlates to the information that is required for the biofeedback device that the author uses. It may vary from device to device but is usually along the same lines. Each practitioner will have their own way of creating a health form to suit their own needs.

Once the information and the hair sample have been programmed into the device it is then ready to begin the test.

How Food Categories are Classified in the Database for Food Sensitivity Testing

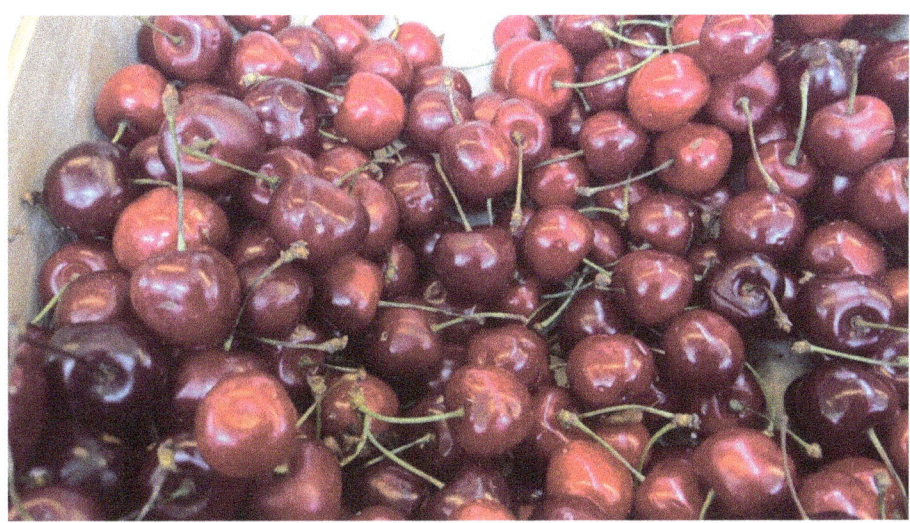

Each device will have its own way of working and usually a pre-programmed database of foods. This database, which is already programmed with a number of foods listed, may well need adding to. There may be a need to add foods from different cultures as we live in a multi-cultural society and also our food is imported from all over the world. If the device has a list of say, 200 foods, then this is a good starting point but there may well be a need to add to this when looking and studying what is needed to give a thorough test.

Here are some lists of foods in the database of the author's own biofeedback device:

(MARS lll)

Diet and Nutrition
Cocoa (uncooked and chocolate bean)
Chocolate
Cereal or Grain products
Barley
Bread, wholemeal
Bread, white bread
Buckwheat
Cornflakes
Maize flour
Millet
Noodles
Porridge oats
Quinoa
Rice
Rye
Sesame
Soya
Spelt
Pasta
Wheat
Wheat, ground
Wheat, wholegrain
Dairy products
Butter
Butter (salted)
Buttermilk
Cheese
Blue Cheese
Soft Cheese
Hard Cheese
Cream Cheese
Cottage Cheese
Cream
Feta
Goat's cheese

Milk
Milk (sour)
Milk (sweet)
Rice milk
Yoghurt
Soya Milk
Drinks
Beer
Chocolate
Cocoa
Coffee (black)
Coffee white
Coffee (with sugar)
Cola
Fruit Juices
Fruit Squash
Fruit Teas
Gin
Ovaltine
Rum (red)
Rum (white)
Tea black
Tea (green)
Tea white
Whisky
Wine (general)
Vodka
Fats, general
Cod liver oil
Oils, general
Olive oil
Peppermint oil
Vegetable fat
Vegetable oil
Fruit Cooked
Apples
Apricots
Blueberries
Blackberries

Cherries
Cranberries
Gooseberries
Grapefruit
Peaches
Pineapples
Plums
Quince
Raisins
Raspberries
Strawberries
Fruit Raw
Apples
Apricots
Avocado
Bananas
Blueberries
Blackberries
Blackcurrants
Cherries
Currents (red, black etc)
Dates
Figs
Gooseberries
Kiwis
Grapefruit
Grapes (red)
Grapes (white)
Honeydew melon
Lychees
Lemons
Limes
Oranges
Papaya
Peaches
Pears
Plums, Damsons
Pomegranates
Prunes
Raisins
Raspberries

Strawberries
Water-melon
Pink Grapefruit
Meat
Bacon
Beef
Beef, dried
Chicken
Chicken, capon
Duck
Duck, domestic
Duck, wild
Egg
Egg white
Egg yolk
Goat
Goose
Wild Boar
Ham
Lamb
Liver (lamb)
Liver
Liver (pig)
Mutton
Pork
Rabbit
Pheasant
Turkey
Veal
Venison
Metabolism
Acid
Carbohydrates
Enzymes
Fats
Glucose
Glycerine
Proteins
Sugar balance (regulation)

Nuts
Almond
Brazil nuts
Cashew nuts
Chestnuts
Coconut
Ground nuts
Hazel nuts
Peanuts
Pecan nuts
Walnuts
Seeds
Pumpkin
Sunflower
Sesame
Seafood/fish
Clams
Cod
Crayfish
Eel
Fish (general)
Fish (general, fresh water)
Fish (general, salt water)
Halibut
Herring
Herring (red)
Lobster
Mackerel
Mussel, common
Mussels, general
Oyster
Plaice
Salmon
Smoked Salmon
Sardine
Shellfish
Shrimp
Potted Shrimps
Smoked herring, bloater
Sole

Trout (brown)
Trout (sea)
Whitefish
Winkles
Spices
Acetic acid
Aniseed
Cinnamon
Cumin
Curry
Ginger
Horse radish
Nutmeg
Paprika
Pepper (black)
Pepper (green)
Pepper (red)
Pepper (white)
Rosemary
Sage
Salt
Thyme
Turmeric
Vinegar (clear)
Vinegar (malt)
Yeast
Sweeteners
Confectionery, general
Honey
Maple
Molasses
Rock candy
Sugar
Sugar, Brown (natural)
Sugar, white
White (industrial sugar)
Vegetables (cooked)
Artichoke
Asparagus

Aubergine
Beans (broad)
Beans (green)
Beans, lima
Beans, navy
Beets
Cabbage
Capsicum (green)
Capsicum (red)
Capsicum (yellow)
Carrots
Cauliflower – fennel
Celery
Courgettes
Garlic
Leek
Lentils
Maize
Mushrooms
Mustard (green)
Okra
Onion
Peas
Peas (field)
Potatoes
Rice
Spinach
Swede
Tomato
Turnip
Vegetable (raw)
Artichoke
Avocado
Broad beans
Brussel Sprouts
Cabbage
Carrots
Cauliflower
Celery
Cress
Garlic

Head lettuce
Olives (black)
Olives (green)
Onions
Parsley
Radish
Scarlet runner beans
Swede
Tomatoes
Watercress

It may be necessary to add to this list and most devices will allow this to be done easily. The foods are broken down into categories between, meat, fish, fruits, vegetables, grains and so on. There is a function that allows there to be different and specialised food tests such as the 'wheat and gluten', 'dairy and lactose' or the 'fruit' tests. The foods are broken down into categories to make it easier for the practitioner to develop their own specialised way of working. For some practitioners may have an interest in Diabetes for example, so they may wish to develop their own 'sugar test' for fast-releasing sugars. This is done by way of creating a new template.

Chapter 8

Health Conditions often associated with Food Sensitivities – Understanding the difference between Food Sensitivities, Intolerances and Allergies

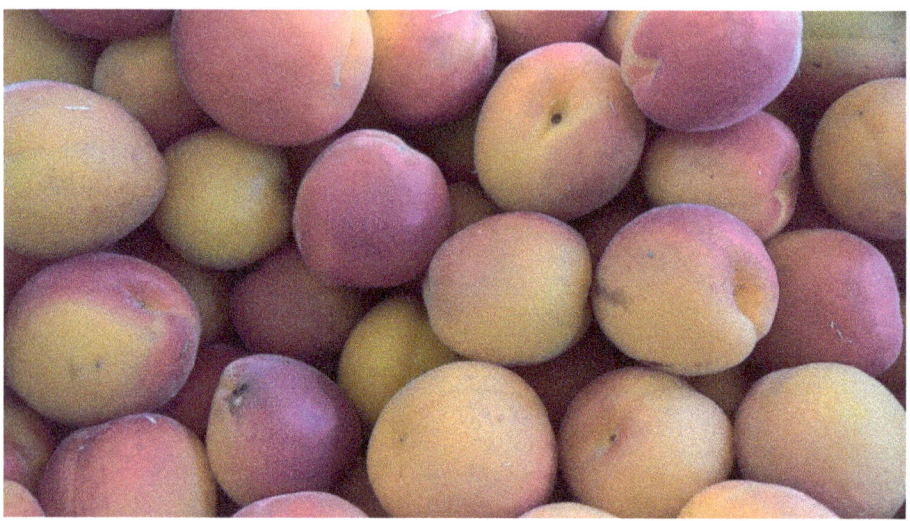

Obesity
Overweight and obesity are defined as abnormal or excessive fat accumulation that may impair health.
Body mass index (BMI) is a simple index of weight-for-height that is commonly used to classify overweight and obesity in adults. It is defined as a person's weight in kilogrammes divided by the square of his height in metres (kg/m2).

Adults
For adults, World Health Organisation defines overweight and obesity as follows:
- overweight is a BMI greater than or equal to 25; and
- obesity is a BMI greater than or equal to 30.

(Source: World Health Organisation –
http://www.who.int/mediacentre/factsheets/fs311/en/)

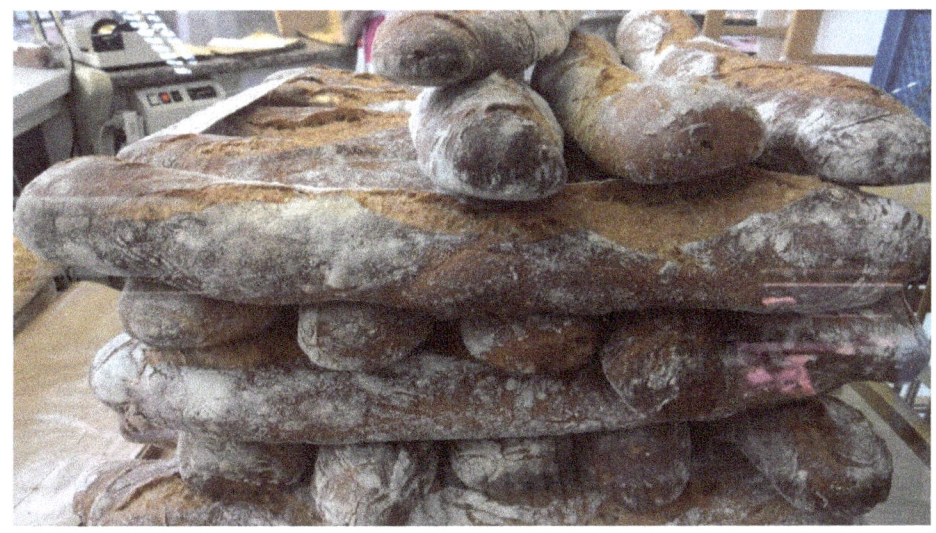

Hypoglycaemia

Hypoglycaemia, or a "hypo", is an abnormally low level of glucose in your blood (less than four millimoles per litre). When your glucose (sugar) level is too low, your body doesn't have enough energy to carry out its activities.

Hypoglycaemia is most commonly associated with diabetes, and mainly occurs if someone with diabetes takes too much insulin, misses a meal or exercises too hard.
(Source: NHS Choices – http://www.nhs.uk/Conditions/Hypoglycaemia/Pages/Introduction.aspx)

Anorexia Nervosa

Anorexia nervosa is a psychological and possibly life-threatening eating disorder defined by an extremely low body weight relative to stature, extreme and needless weight loss, illogical fear of weight gain, and distorted perception of self-image and body. This is called Body Mass Index (BMI) and is a function of an individual's height and weight.
Additionally, women and men who suffer from anorexia nervosa exemplify a fixation with a thin figure and abnormal eating patterns. Anorexia nervosa is interchangeable with the term anorexia, which refers to self-starvation and lack of appetite.

Examples of biological factors include:

- Irregular hormone functions

- Genetics (the tie between anorexia and one's genes is still being heavily researched, but we know that genetics is a part of the story).
- Nutritional deficiencies.

(Source: https://www.eatingdisorderhope.com/information/anorexia#What-is-Anorexia)

Bulimia Nervosa

Bulimia nervosa is a psychological and severe life-threatening eating disorder described by the ingestion of an abnormally large amount of food in a short time period, followed by an attempt to avoid gaining weight by purging what was consumed.

Methods of purging include forced vomiting, excessive use of laxatives or diuretics, and extreme or prolonged periods of exercising.

Symptoms include:
- Constant weight fluctuations.
- Electrolyte imbalances, which can result in cardiac arrhythmia, cardiac arrest, or ultimately death.
- Broken blood vessels within the eyes.
- Enlarged glands in the neck and under the jawline.
- Oral trauma, such as lacerations in the lining of the mouth or throat from repetitive vomiting.
- Chronic dehydration.
- Inflammation of the oesophagus.
- Chronic gastric reflux after eating or peptic ulcers.
- Infertility.

(Source: https://www.eatingdisorderhope.com/information/bulimia)

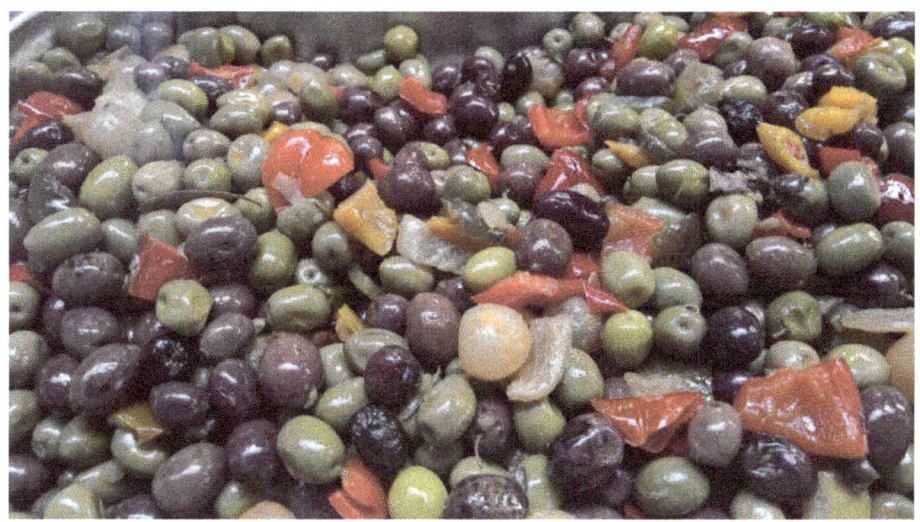

Candida Albicans

Candida albicans is an opportunistic fungus (or form of yeast) that is the cause of candida related complex and many undesirable symptoms including fatigue, weight gain, joint pain, and gas. The candida albicans yeast is a normal part of your gut flora, a group of microorganisms that live in your digestive tract.

Most people have some level of candida albicans in their intestines, and usually it coexists peacefully with the other bacteria and yeasts that live there. But a combination of factors can lead to the candida albicans population getting out of control, establishing fast-growing colonies and biofilms, and starting to dominate your gut.

At this point it can begin to affect your digestion, weaken your immune system, and even damage your intestinal wall, penetrating through into the bloodstream and releasing its toxic by-products throughout your body.

As they spread, these toxic by-products cause damage to your body tissues and organs, wreaking havoc on your health and wellbeing. The major waste product of yeast cell activity is acetaldehyde, a poisonous neurotoxin that promotes free radical activity in the body. Acetaldehyde is usually broken down into acetic acid within the liver. However, if this process is not working efficiently, or too much acetaldehyde is being released, then it can circulate through your body and cause unpleasant symptoms like headaches and nausea.
(Source: https://www.thecandidadiet.com/what-is-candida-albicans/)

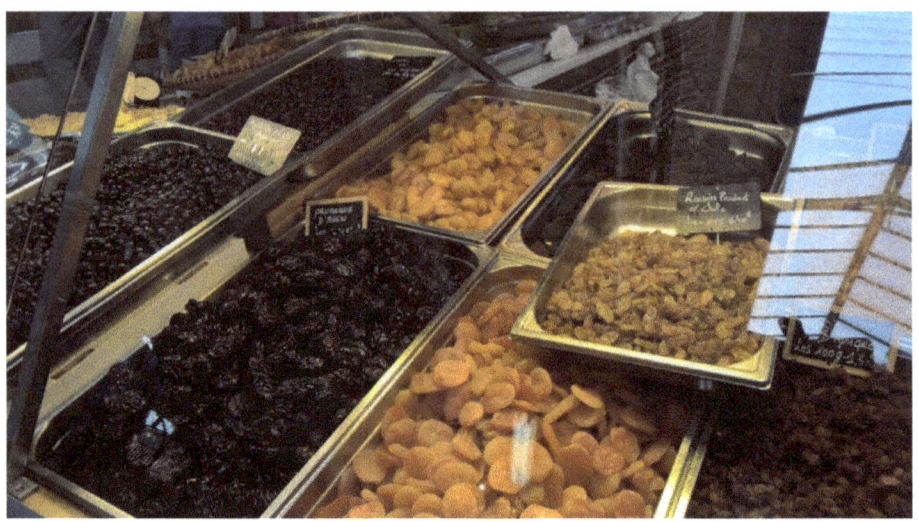

Diabetes

Type 1 diabetes develops if the body can't produce enough insulin, because insulin-producing cells in the pancreas have been destroyed. It can happen:
- Because of genetic factors.
- When a virus or infection triggers an autoimmune response (where the body starts attacking itself).

People who have this type of diabetes are usually diagnosed before they're forty and there's currently no way to prevent it. It's the least common type of diabetes – only 10% of all cases are type 14.

Type 2 diabetes develops when the body can still make some insulin, but not enough, or when the body becomes resistant to insulin. It can happen:
- When people are overweight and inactive. People who are an 'apple-shape' (with lots of fat around the abdomen) have a greater risk of developing type 2 diabetes.
- Because of genetic factors.

People who have this type of diabetes are usually diagnosed when they're over forty, and it's more common in men. However, more overweight children and young people in the UK are being diagnosed with the condition. It is also particularly common among people of African-Caribbean, Asian and Hispanic origin, and 90% of all adults with diabetes have type 2 diabetes.

Being extremely tired, blurred vision and feeling more thirsty than usual are all symptoms associated with diabetes. Some additional signs of undiagnosed diabetes can include:
- Going to the toilet to urinate more often than usual, especially at night.
- Unexplained weight loss, genital itching or regular episodes of thrush.
- Slow healing of cuts and wounds.
- Unexplained weight loss.

With type 1 diabetes, signs and symptoms are usually obvious and develop very quickly over a few weeks. Once the diabetes is treated and under control, symptoms will go away quickly.

In type 2 diabetes, signs and symptoms may not be so obvious. The condition develops slowly over several years, and it might only be picked up in a routine medical check-up. As with type 1 diabetes, symptoms are quickly relieved once diabetes is treated and under control.
(Source: https://www.drinkaware.co.uk)

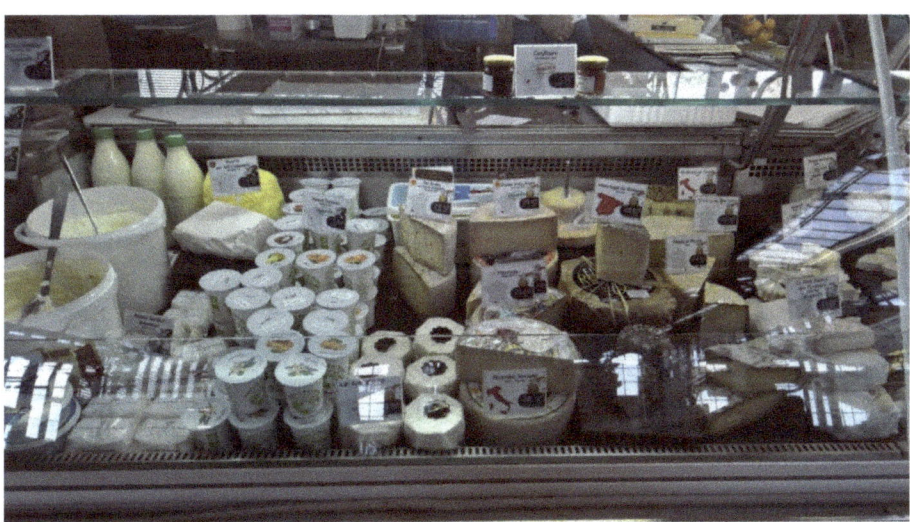

Irritable Bowel Syndrome
Irritable bowel syndrome (IBS) is a common, long-term condition of the digestive system. It can cause bouts of stomach cramps, bloating, diarrhoea and/or constipation.
Some of the reasons contributing towards IBS are as follows:
- Foods or drinks that trigger your symptoms.
- The amount of fibre in your diet.
- Stress.

It may help to:
- Exercise regularly.
- Reduce your stress levels.
- Test for food sensitivities.

(Source: http://www.nhs.uk/Conditions/Irritable-bowel-syndrome/Pages/Introduction.aspx)

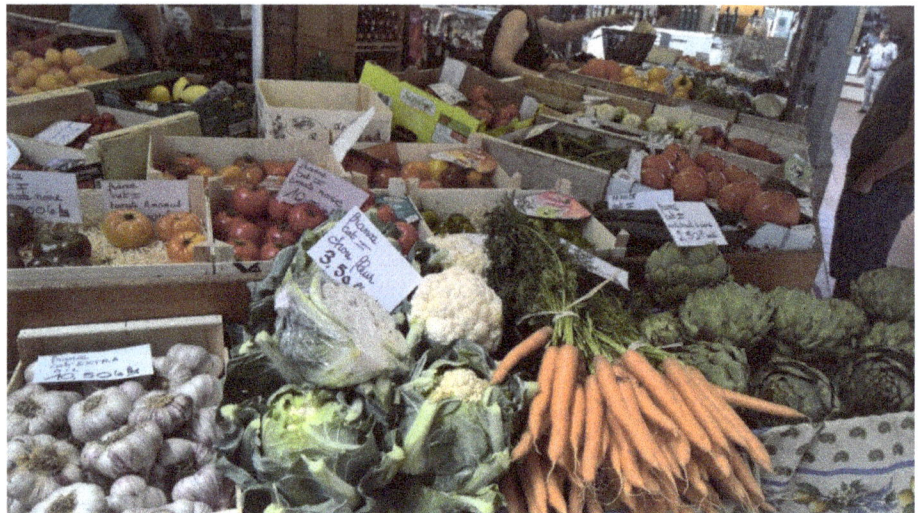

Stress and Anxiety

The difference between them is that stress is a response to a threat in a situation. Anxiety is a reaction to the stress. Chronic stress can affect your health, causing symptoms from headaches, high blood pressure, and chest pain to heart palpitations, skin rashes, and loss of sleep.

(Source: https://www.adaa.org/understanding-anxiety/related-illnesses/ stress)

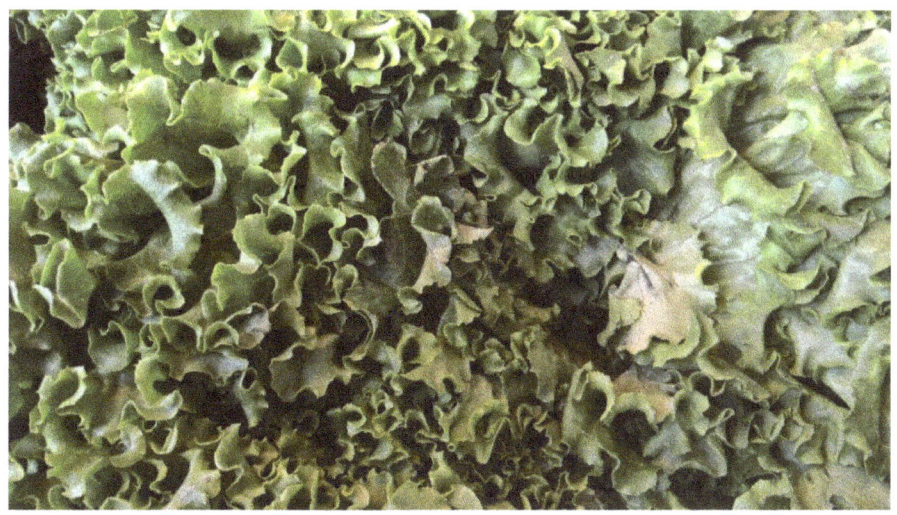

Pre Menstrual Syndrome (PMT)

Premenstrual syndrome (PMS) is the name given to the physical, psychological and behavioural symptoms that can occur in the two weeks before a woman's monthly period. It's also known as premenstrual tension (PMT).

There are many different symptoms of PMS, but typical examples are:
- Bloating.
- Breast pain.
- Mood swings.
- Feeling irritable.
- Loss of interest in sex.

It may help to do the following:
- A healthy diet.
- Regular exercise to improve your health and fitness.
- Learning techniques to help relieve stress.
- Regular sleep.

(Source: http://www.nhs.uk/conditions/premenstrual-syndrome/pages/introduction.aspx)

Asthma

Symptoms of asthma include:
- Shortness of breath.
- Wheezing – making a noise like a whistle when you breathe out.

- Tightness in the chest.
- Coughing.

Triggers:
- The common cold.
- Allergies to things like pollen and animal fur and certain foods.
- Irritants, like tobacco smoke, spray cleaners and dust.
- Heightened emotions.
- Air pollution especially from traffic.

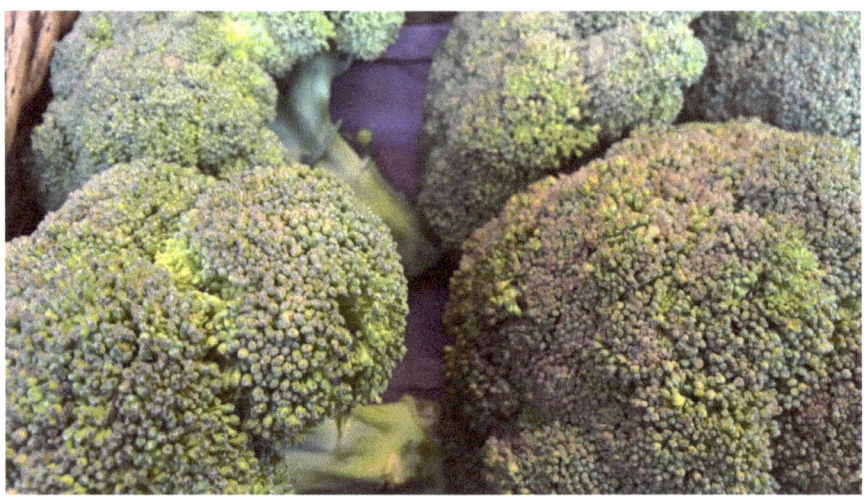

Skin Conditions
- Eczema – cracked, dry, itchy sore skin.
- Dermatitis – as above.
- Psoriasis – flaky red sore skin that can be itchy.
- Cold Sores – small blisters caused by the herpes simplex virus.
- Hives (urticaria) – raised itchy rash.
- Impetigo – infectious sores.

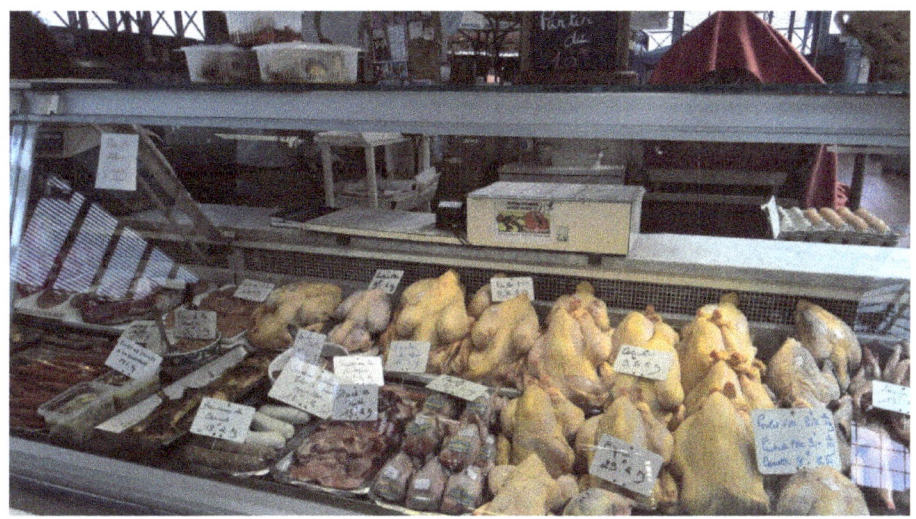

Diarrhoea and Constipation
Diarrhoea is usually due to a bowel infection caused by a pathogen or food sensitivity; constipation is usually caused by poor diet, insufficient fluid intake, stress, alcohol consumption of food sensitivities

Cystitis
Cystitis is inflammation of the bladder, and can be caused by infection or insufficient fluid intake together with straining to pass stools. It is also thought to be involved in a yeast infection such as Candida.

Thrush
Thrush is a yeast infection or overgrowth which can cause itching in the vaginal area including the internal vaginal canal.

Migraine
Migraine is a severe headache that can cause throbbing pain and visual disturbances as well as a feeling of nausea. In some cases vomiting does occur. Triggers can be alcohol, stress, fatigue, inadequate sleep, food intolerances, hormones and computer screens.

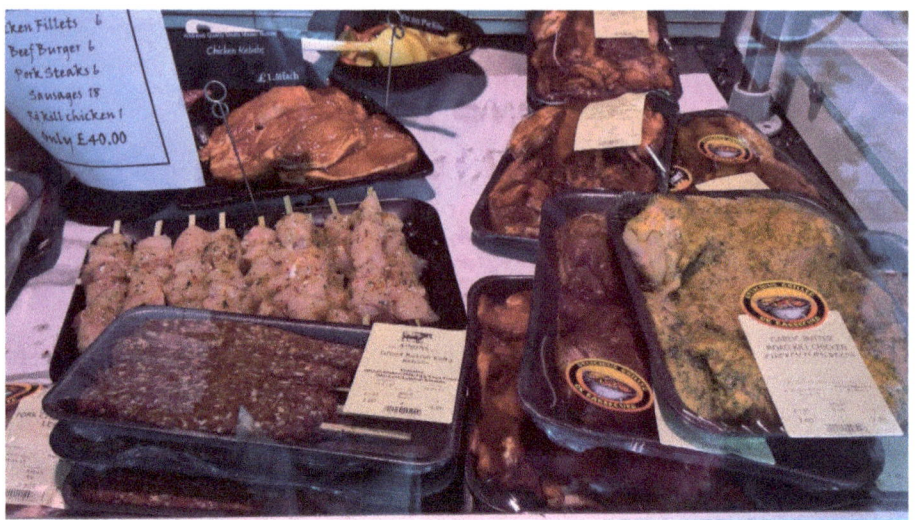

Insomnia
This is caused by a lack of sleep due to the inability to sleep. This can be caused by medications, alcohol, stress and worry, environmental factors and lifestyle.

Fatigue
Tiredness is often caused by mental or physical over-exertion or illness, creating a feeling of exhaustion. Foods can also be involved in this feeling of fatigue by depleting the body of essential nutrients for vitality.

What is understood by the terms food allergies, food sensitivities and food intolerances:

Allergies
A food allergy is defined by a severe acute reaction to a specific food; this may cause swelling of the tongue, lips and respiratory organs, rapid heart rate, dizziness, skin rash and/or change of skin colour, shaking, upset stomach/sickness or fainting. This can be very frightening and serious. This also means that this food should never be eaten.

Sensitivities
Food sensitivities are mainly defined by the symptoms such as bloating, excessive gas, indigestion, irritable bowel (IBS), loose stools, lethargy, tiredness after eating, skin sensitivities such as dry skin/sore skin, psoriasis, blocked sinuses or excessive mucous and sometimes weight gain. Food sensitivities may cause chronic and long-term health symptoms if not addressed. This indicates that a certain food or food group may need

to be avoided for a while before it can be reintroduced to identify whether this is a long-term sensitivity or food intolerance.

Intolerances

The food sensitivity test is designed to help identify food sensitivities. However, if subsequent food tests indicate the same food sensitivities each time, it is highly likely that this food becomes a food intolerance, which means that it is best left out of the diet long term.

Allergy or Intolerance?

A food allergy is where the body's immune system reacts to a specific food. The body releases antibodies called immunoglobulin E (IgE) in response to the allergen. The antibodies then move to certain cells where chemicals are released. It is this release of chemicals that causes the allergic reaction. Many symptoms can occur such as itching, swelling or rashes. Common allergens are peanuts, shellfish, eggs, milk, pollen and insect bites.

This specific response of an allergy is different to a food intolerance or sensitivity. A food intolerance or food sensitivity is generally less severe and is associated with the body's inability to digest the food. The immune system is not triggered by food intolerance. Some of the common intolerances include wheat and dairy; general digestive discomfort such as bloating, diarrhoea and nausea are all typical responses to food intolerance.

Chapter 9

Nutrition

Outline of Foods and Nutritional Information including diagrams of the Digestive System

This part of the manual explains the role that nutrition plays in overall health. This gives the practitioner some practical knowledge with food composition, diet and food sensitivities, intolerances and allergies. This knowledge is essential for any practitioner working with food sensitivities.

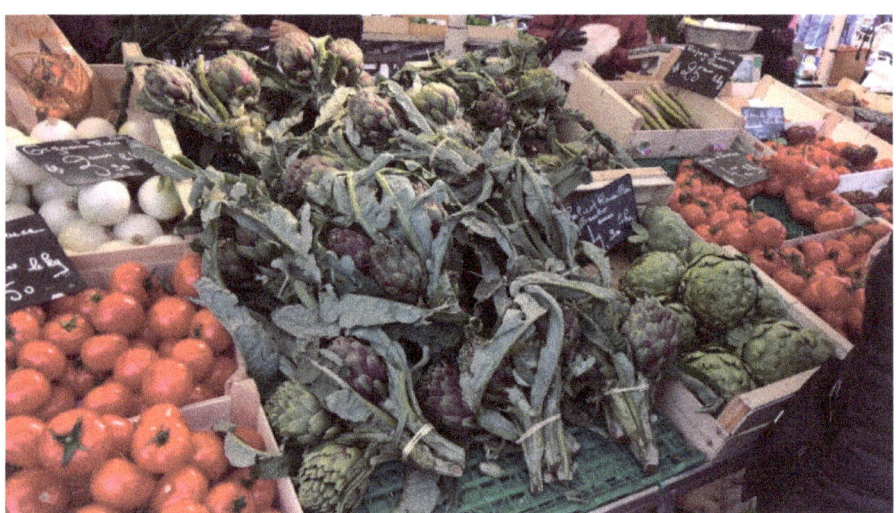

Diet and Nutrition
Fundamentally nutrition is essential for our health. Nutrition refers to the study of the nourishment through food. Our cells depend upon nutrition for our growth, maintenance, repair and metabolism. We obtain nutrients through food sources in either a solid or liquid state and within these foods are nutrients such as protein, carbohydrates, essential fats, vitamins, minerals and water. It is through the balance of these nutrients within our diets that the body is able to function at its best. Without adequate nutrition, the body is likely to be susceptible to diseases and delayed growth.

Diet is the particular intake consumed by an individual. It might be beneficial to analyse how diets change from person to person? There are many influencing factors such as culture or religious beliefs that can vary a person's diet. There may be other factors that influence a person's diet such as specific health conditions. Conditions such as Type 2 Diabetes can be controlled by diet alone.

The Digestive System

After food is ingested it begins on a long journey through the digestive system, which in total covers over 30ft. It can take the food a day to cover the course of muscular tubes and chambers. Once we ingest the food substance it is broken down in the mouth through chewing. Salivary glands help to break down the food too. Saliva contains a digestive enzyme called amylase (salivary amylase), which begins the breakdown of starches and salts. The saliva also helps to lubricate the food, making swallowing and chewing easier. It also helps to keep the mouth moist and comfortable between eating. The food then continues down the pharynx though the oesophagus to the stomach. The stomach not only breaks the food into small particles but secretes digestive enzymes to help break the food down. These include pepsin, which is the main gastric enzyme as it breaks proteins into smaller particles. Other enzymes in the stomach are gelatinase, gastric amylase and gastric lipase.

The pancreas helps the process as it also produces enzymes. The pancreas is the main digestive gland in the body. These juices include alkalis that neutralize the stomach acid and roughly fifteen enzymes which work on carbohydrates, proteins and fats. These include trypsin that breaks down peptides in the small intestine and steapsin, which changes triglycerides into fatty acids and glycerol.

By the time the food and enzymes reach the duodenum, most of the food particles are very small though not small enough to pass through the membranes and into the body's tissues. The broken-down part liquid mass known as chyme (partially digested food) then passes into the small intestine where a chemical process breaks down the food into very small molecules. This helps it to pass into the bloodstream. The chyme is released at intervals into the small intestine. Further digestive enzymes are released in the small intestine such as lactase and maltase that help to break down sugars. Lactase breaks down lactose into glucose and galactose and maltase breaks down maltose into glucose. There is also the enzyme sucrase in the small intestine, which breaks down sucrose into glucose and fructose. These enzymes act within the lining cells and on their surfaces. What is left and is unable to pass into the bloodstream is compacted within the large intestine as faeces. The faeces pass through the anus to be expelled.

Food is able to be passed through the digestive system due to the muscular contractions of the body. These contractions are known as peristalsis.

The Role of Water within our Body

Water is essential for every form of life. It is a compound of hydrogen and oxygen and is also referred to as H_2O. Two hydrogen atoms attach to a single oxygen atom in each molecule of water. Although the human body can last weeks without food it can only function a few days without water. Water makes up two thirds of an adult's body weight. To remain hydrated in the UK one would need to drink 1.2 litres (6 to 8 glasses) of water or fluid a day to maintain the balance and prevent dehydration. In hotter countries or with more activity this amount would need to increase.

Water is vital for our body's growth and maintenance and is essential for our cells. All living cells within our body require a moist internal environment. It is a major participant of all the chemical reactions that occur both within and outside of our body's cells. 60% of our body's water is contained within the cells and both the spaces between cells (intercellular spaces) and the spaces inside cells (intracellular spaces) are filled with water. Our total body water is made up of intracellular fluid at 40% and extracellular fluid at 20% making a total of 60% of our body weight.

Water helps us with bodily functions such as to regulate temperature and the moistening of food. It also dilutes waste products and poisonous substances from the body. It also transports substances within our bodies such as nutrients and hormones and oxygen to our cells. Water is also essential for providing the medium of excretion of waste products such as urine and faeces from the body. Approximately 90% of our blood consists of water and therefore it is an essential part of blood and tissue fluid. It also protects our organs and joints by acting as a lubricant.

Without enough water our bodies can become dehydrated. Causes of dehydration can be increased exercise or a change in climate as water is lost from the body in the form of sweat. Vomiting and diarrhoea can also lead to dehydration. Dehydration can cause headaches, joint pain, tiredness and constipation. Severe dehydration can lead to kidney stones and severe confusion.

Carbohydrates, Fats and Proteins

Carbohydrates can be classified into three main groups: sugars, starches and non-starch polysaccharides. Sugars and starches are an essential source of food energy for our bodies. Monosaccharides provide 3.75 kcal per gram and disaccharides 4 kcal per gram.

Glucose is the main source of energy for all of the cells of the body. It is also needed for an energy source for the brain and for the red blood cells. Without carbohydrates our bodies would be unable to function well. Without any carbohydrate the body would resort to breaking down fat and muscle to obtain an energy supply.

Non-starch polysaccharide, known as fibre, is essential to our digestive system as it aids in the excretion of waste products from our bodies. Without sufficient fibre, constipation could occur leading to a build-up of toxins and can lead to other diseases. Soluble fibre dissolves in water and forms a gel that slows down the digestion and absorption of carbohydrates. It lowers cholesterol, which can help prevent heart disease and helps to control blood glucose levels.

Insoluble fibre adds bulk to the stool helping it to move quickly through the digestive tract. This helps reduce the risk of colon cancer and constipation.

Fats are a compound of oxygen, carbon and hydrogen. Fats are a much more concentrated form of energy to carbohydrates. The energy obtained is double in fat to an equal weight of carbohydrate or protein.

When found in food, fat is a mixture of triglycerides. Each of the triglycerides is one unit of glycerol and three fatty acids. Different combinations of these make up different types of fats or oils. They differ in the number of carbon atoms they contain and the amount of hydrogen atoms that the carbon atoms hold.

Saturated fatty acids are considered stable as they have as many hydrogen atoms that they can hold. Carbon atoms form different bonds when there are hydrogen atoms missing. Monounsaturated fatty acids contain two double bonds. This means that it is missing two hydrogen atoms. Polyunsaturated fatty acids have two or more double bonds meaning that there are at least four hydrogen atoms missing. These react with oxygen to make rancid fat when left exposed.

Trans fats are fats that contain trans unsaturated fatty acids. These occur in dairy produce and the flesh of meat.

Fats can be found in both animal and vegetable sources. Vegetable sources include seeds such as peanuts and coconuts and vegetable seeds, which are a good source of omega 6 polyunsaturated fatty acids. Animal sources include fish, which is a source of omega 3 polyunsaturated fatty acids and meats such as beef, lamb and pork.

Some polyunsaturated fats include linoleic acid and alpha-linolenic acid. These were originally called vitamin F. These are essential fatty acids because they cannot be made in the body. Some polyunsaturated fats are found in plant and fish oils. One of these is gamma linolenic acid.

The energy obtained in fat is double that to an equal weight of carbohydrate or protein.

Fats can provide the body with a reserve supply of energy when the carbohydrate energy supply runs out. Some animal fats contain vitamins such as A (retinol) and vitamin D and some vegetable fats contain vitamin E and carotenes that can be converted to retinol by the body. These vitamins cannot be absorbed without the presence of fat in our bodies. Cholesterol is also found in animal fat, which is essential to our bodies for cell membranes.

Fats also help to flavour and add texture certain foods and provides us with insulation under the skin. Too little fat results in dry, flaky skin. It also helps to cushion and protect some of our organs such as the heart and is part of the membrane that surrounds our cells. This helps the cells to function properly.

Fats are also main components of hormones. Too much of trans unsaturated fatty acids found in vegetable oils can lead to an increased risk of heart disease and a high level of blood cholesterol. Saturated fatty acids found in dairy foods and animal produce also has the same effect on the body. Smoking can also cause high cholesterol and an increased risk of heart disease.

It is recommended that an adult's total fat intake should not be more than 35% of dietary energy. Of that 35%, only 10% should be of saturated fat. It is also recommended that omega 6 polyunsaturated fatty acids provide 6% of the energy.

Proteins are essential for the body's growth and repair. Any excess can be converted to glucose in the liver and used for energy by the body. Proteins are made up of amino acids. Non-essential amino acids can be made by the body and essential amino acids cannot be made by the body but have to be obtained from food.

The essential amino acids are tryptophan, valine, leucine, isoleucine, methionine, phenylalanine, threonine and lysine. These amino acids cannot be made by the body and therefore need to be taken in through food sources. If a food source contains all of these eight amino acids it is classed as a complete protein. There are two amino acids that are essential for infants: histidine and taurine.

The remaining non-essential amino acids are alanine, arginine, aspartic acid, asparagine, cysteine, glutamic acid, glutamine, glycine, proline, serine and tyrosine. These amino acids can all be made by the body by the excess of other amino acids taken in by the body. Amino acids can be found in proteins such as fish, meat, eggs, soya and quinoa.

Our cells are constantly regenerating and protein is necessary for the replacement of worn-out cells and for tissue repair. The proteins produce antibodies which help fight the bacteria, viruses, toxins and other foreign substances that are harmful to the body. Therefore it helps in the healing process of our cells.

Protein is necessary for our growth throughout our life. Babies absorb protein from their mother's milk.

1.1 Which categories do the following foods fall into?

	Carbohydrates	Fats	Proteins
Grains			
Vegetables			
Beans and Pulses			
Pasta			
Fruit			
Sweets			
Milk			
Cheese			
Oil			
Oily Fish			

Carbohydrate can include grains, vegetables, beans, pasta, fruit, sugary cakes and sweets; proteins can includes meat, fish, cheese, eggs, nuts and broccoli, and fats can include dairy, avocados, oily fish, oils, nuts and seeds.

Sugar
Refined sugar undergoes a process called refining by which the sucrose is extracted from the plant and then the parts of the plant that are not wanted such as the stalk fibres, bacteria, insect debris and moulds are removed. The carbohydrate that is left contains very little minerals. To make white

sugar, bleaching agents are then added. The sugar is then refined further by being filtered in a liquid state (by water being added) through beef bone char. The finished state of the sugar is 99.9% sucrose and contains no nutritional elements. It is also referred to as empty calories. Refined sugar can have a negative effect on the body and cause conditions such as obesity, tooth decay and diabetes.

Unrefined sugar is made from the juice of the sugar cane plant. Unlike refined sugar it contains trace minerals and nutrients. These include calcium, magnesium, iron, potassium and phosphorus. Unrefined sugar does not contain any of the harmful chemicals such as phosphoric acid, sulphur dioxide that are added to refined sugar.

Processed sugar can have many harmful effects on the body. Excessive sugars can be the cause or contributing factor of many conditions, and organs can be affected or compromised due to excessive sugar intake. Too much sugar can cause the body to become too acidic and as a result the body takes nutrients from its reserves leaving less. One of the minerals used to neutralise high acidity in the cells is calcium. The body would eventually take calcium from the bones and teeth. There is also the danger of osteoporosis and arthritic conditions arising.

Excess sugar can lead to weight gain. The liver can only store a certain amount of sugar. When the liver has reached its full capacity the excess glucose is returned to the body in the form of fat. Fat deposits are then distributed around the body such as the hips, buttocks and stomach. Eventually the fatty deposits become stored around major organs such as the heart when the more inactive parts of the body are full. This can be incredibly damaging and lead to poor function and a deterioration of these organs.

Sugar also affects the immune system as it can result in a lower amount of white blood cells, which are essential for fighting infections and disease. Increased sugar intake also increases the production of adrenaline. It stimulates the flight of fight response. This response increases the production of cortisone which suppresses immune function. The flight of fight response gives us a false feeling of energy; only in truth once this response has worn off, the body experiences a feeling of a crash and energy levels hit a low. Insomnia can also be experienced.

Diabetes is a condition that can occur from a diet high in sugar. Sufferers find it difficult to metabolise their blood sugar. Imbalances of blood sugar levels can result in glaucoma, kidney diseases, high blood pressure and anxiety. Constant monitoring of this disease is essential.

Gum disease and tooth decay are other problems associated with consuming excess amounts of sugar.

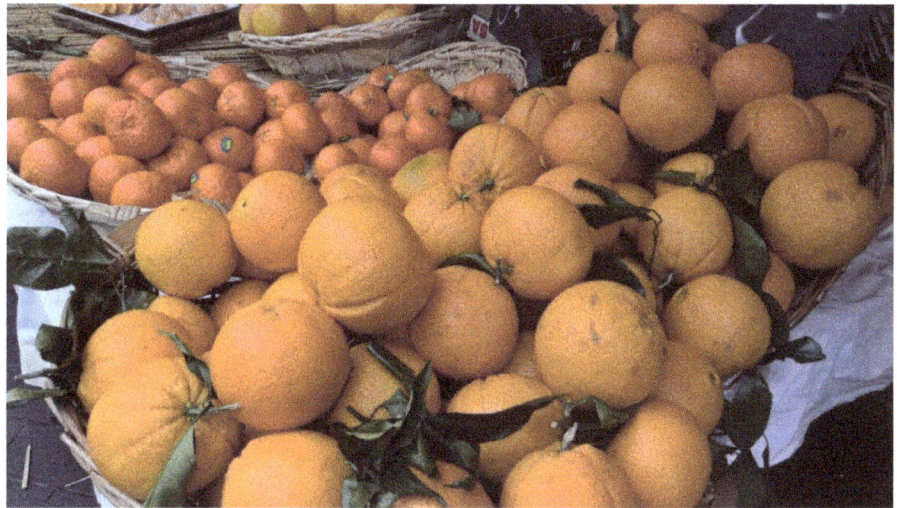

The glycaemic index is the figure to establish how much blood sugar will be raised after eating a carbohydrate food. The lower the number the less of an impact the food will have on the person's glucose level. The rating scores from 0–100. A reading of 100 would indicate the substance to be pure glucose.

Foods such as sugar, sweets, fizzy drinks, white bread and white potatoes are all broken down quickly in the body and cause the blood glucose to rise quickly. Therefore these foods are known to be of a high GI rating. Foods such as vegetables, some fruits, wholegrain foods and pulses are either medium or low GI foods.

Foods digest differently depending on what they are consumed with. Carbohydrates are absorbed slower when eaten with fat or protein. Mixing a high GI food and a low GI food equals a medium GI rating.

The GI diet is useful for diabetics to ensure they do not eat foods that will cause a blood sugar low (hypoglycaemia) such as high GI foods. Once the blood sugar level has risen rapidly it subsequently falls, causing the blood glucose level to drop. By combining foods they can delay absorption and even out blood glucose levels.

Fibre
Fibre is essential to our digestive system as it aids in the excretion of waste products from our bodies. Without sufficient fibre, constipation can be present leading to an accumulation of toxins which can lead to other diseases.

Soluble fibre is found in fruits, vegetables, beans, oats, barley, potatoes, lentils, dried fruit and soya products. Soluble fibre dissolves in water and forms a gel that slows down the digestion and absorption of carbohydrates. It lowers cholesterol which can help prevent heart disease and helps to control blood glucose levels.

Insoluble fibre is found in vegetables, whole grains, wholemeal flour, brown rice, some fruits and wholemeal pasta. It adds bulk to the stool helping it to move quickly through the digestive tract. This helps reduce the risk of colon cancer and constipation.

Food can have a big impact on varying health conditions and diseases. These are a few conditions that food may play a significant role in:

Heart Disease
Heart disease can be caused by excessive cholesterol in the blood. High levels of low density protein can be deposited on the walls of blood vessels. As this 'plaque' builds, it narrows the arteries restricting blood flow. If the blood supply is severely blocked then a heart attack or death can occur.

High levels of LDL are contributed to by a diet high in saturated fat. Saturated fat content is high in foods such as butter, margarine and cocoa butter.

Omega 3 polyunsaturated fatty acids may help to prevent heart disease by ensuring that the heart cell membranes are stable and by decreasing the probability of the blood clotting. Foods rich in Omega 3 would be oily fish such as sardines, salmon and mackerel.

High Blood Pressure
High blood pressure can be caused by an excessive alcohol intake and by obesity. An excessively high intake of foods that is not balanced with an individual's energy need results in excess fat being stored in the body. Eating a diet high in saturated fat such as cakes and biscuits and eating fried food can contribute to obesity. High salt intakes have also been linked to high blood pressure. It is advised that an adult should not consume more than 6 grams of salt a day.

Diabetes
Diabetes is a condition that can occur from a diet high in sugar. Sufferers find it difficult to metabolise their blood sugar. Sometimes the pancreas fails to produce any insulin or not enough, which means that the glucose doesn't reach the cells. This is Type 1 diabetes. Type 2 diabetes is where the insulin does not react correctly or the tissues develop a resistance to the effects of insulin. Type 2 diabetes can be helped by weight loss to reduce insulin resistance by a lesser intake of food.

Suffers experience increased thirst, a flushed face, sweating and increased urination during hyperglycaemia (high blood sugar) and mood swings, irritability and weakness with low blood sugar levels (hypoglycaemia).

Any foods high in sugar and particularly refined sugar such as sweets, cakes and fizzy drinks are high risk foods. It is recommended that suffers have a diet low in fat, low in sugars, low in salt, high in fruit and vegetables and high in starchy carbohydrates. Suffers should also eat regular meals and keep an even food intake.

Arthritis
Arthritis is a disease causing inflammation of the joints. There are several types of arthritis. Osteoarthritis, rheumatoid arthritis and psoriatic arthritis are all different types and all result in pain to the sufferer.

There has been much controversy regarding the relationship between certain foods and arthritis. Some sufferers find that dairy products make symptoms worse whilst others say that acidic foods such as fruit make symptoms worse.

The nightshade family of foods are a group that some sufferers choose to avoid. These include white potatoes, tomatoes, peppers and eggplant. As there is no conclusive evidence, each individual needs to find what works for them personally.

Alzheimer's
Approximately 70% of dementia sufferers have Alzheimer's disease. It is recommended that due to their increase of oxidants, an increase of antioxidants such as vitamins A, C, E and beta carotene would be a beneficial supplement to the sufferer. Good sources of these vitamins are fresh fruit and vegetables and oily fish and seeds.

It is also thought that eating foods rich in omega 3 fatty acids such as salmon, tuna and mackerel lowers an individual's risk of developing

Alzheimer's. One belief is that the increased intake of omega 3 foods eases the brain inflammation.

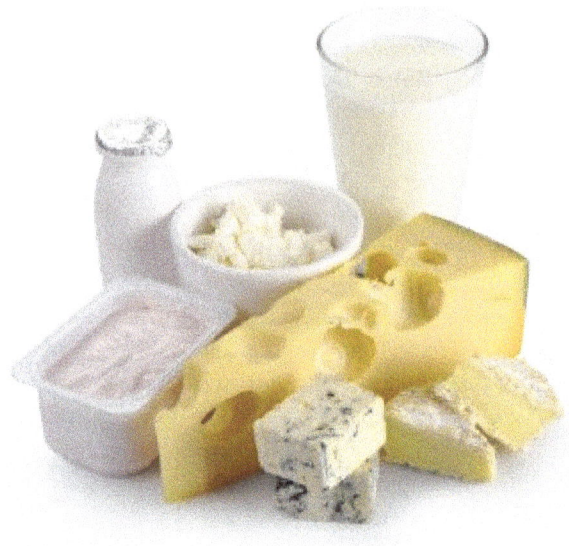

Many foods are now contributing to an increase in both food allergies and food intolerances. There has been a significant increase in nut intolerance over the past few years. Many food factories produce more than one food or meal and 'may contain traces of nuts' is commonly labelled on food packaging as a warning. Most schools now ban nuts in school in any form.

It is unknown as to why there is such an increase in the rise of nut allergy. One possible idea for the rise is that more women consume nuts whilst pregnant and breast feeding. Another theory is that children become sensitised to nuts due to an over exposure of peanut traces in pre-packed food. In extreme cases of nut intolerance, described as a nut allergy, a person can experience an anaphylactic shock which, if not treated, can be fatal. The mouth and tongue rapidly swell after eating the nut and breathing becomes extremely difficult or impossible unless there is medical help.

Thankfully a nut allergy has less severe symptoms. Itching, runny nose, digestive discomfort, tingling of the skin (particularly the mouth) and rashes are a common reaction with this type of allergy.

Babies obtain some protein from their mother's breast milk which contains antibodies, which provide protection from infection. Some children, however, react to certain food proteins called allergens. One of these allergens is nut protein. It is recommended that children under the age of six months are not given any form of nut in case of an allergic reaction.

Peanut allergy is more commonly seen where a family member has an allergic condition such as asthma, eczema or hay fever. It is advised where this is the case that peanuts or any form of peanut-based product such a groundnut oil is not given to the child until the child is at least three years old.

Alternative products might be sunflower, pumpkin or sesame seeds as these all have a similar nutrient value to nuts. Soya is also an alternative and soya beans can be baked into soybeans, which almost resemble a peanut in look, texture and flavour. Other healthy sources of monounsaturated fat are olives and avocados. Avocados are also an excellent source of vitamin E such as peanuts. Another good source of protein and fibre is hummus made from chick peas.

Coeliac disease is a condition in which the sufferer reacts to gluten. Sufferers experience symptoms such as diarrhoea, weight loss, muscle spasms, loss of appetite and abdominal discomfort. The degree and severity of symptoms varies from person to person. If left untreated, malnutrition can occur in severe cases due to a lack of nutrients being absorbed.

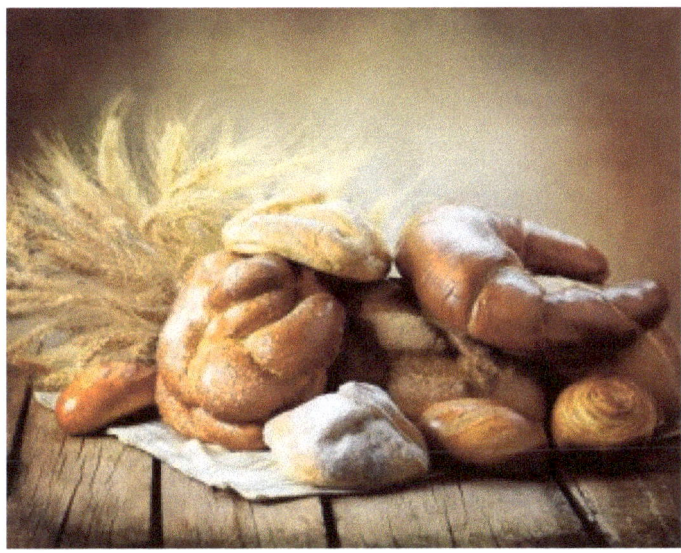

Gluten is produced when water is added to the flour in the preparation of the dough for baking. The proteins gliadin and glutenin combine to form gluten. Once the dough is baked the fermentation stops and the yeast is killed. The gluten holds the pockets of gas and then coagulates as the cooking continues, therefore holding the shape of the bread.

Gluten is most commonly found in foods such as bread and bread products, cakes, cereals, flour, biscuits and noodles. It can also be found in beer, baked beans and gum. The list of foods containing gluten is quite extensive and it is often in foods one would not normally expect.

Many foods are available as gluten free, and those that contain gluten are normally clearly labelled. Most supermarkets have a wide range of gluten-free bread, biscuits, soups, cereal bars and pasta. Rice noodles might be an alternative to pasta. Gluten is not necessary to the health of our bodies and a well-balanced diet can still be maintained by eating gluten-free products.

It is believed that certain food additives may cause changes in behaviour, especially significant in children. These behavioural difficulties include difficulty with learning, memory, sleep disturbance, aggression, mood swings, emotions and language. A food additive is a substance added by the manufacturer to a food or drink in order to either preserve or add colour or flavour. The substance itself is not naturally eaten as a food.

A diet high in carbohydrates is not a balanced diet for anyone and particularly when it includes sweets, cakes and biscuits. Many people believe that this kind of diet causes hyperactivity, mood swings and aggression. This is partly due to their high refined sugar content causing sugar highs and lows, but it is also thought so because of the additives and preservatives added to the food.

A lot of food companies have opted for natural flavourings and preservatives, however, there are many products in our supermarkets that still contain artificial additives and preservatives. There have been many studies done amongst children in the hope of confirming the evidence that additives and E Numbers create hyperactivity; however, to my knowledge, although there are cases where this has proved conclusive it is not a conclusive fact of the medical profession.

One of the E Numbers of particular concern is E211 (Sodium Benzoate). This is found in fizzy drinks and is believed to cause hyperactivity. It is a preservative used to prevent yeast and mould growing. Another is E102 (tartrazine), found in sweets and biscuits which is also linked to hyperactivity. These e-numbers are also said to be linked with medical disorders such as asthma.

The law has now stated that if the following E Numbers listed below are in a food, the label must state that *"the colour may have an adverse effect on activity and attention in children"*.

Sunset yellow (E110), quinoline yellow (E104), carmoisine (E122), allura red (E129), tartrazine (E102) and ponceau 4R (E124).

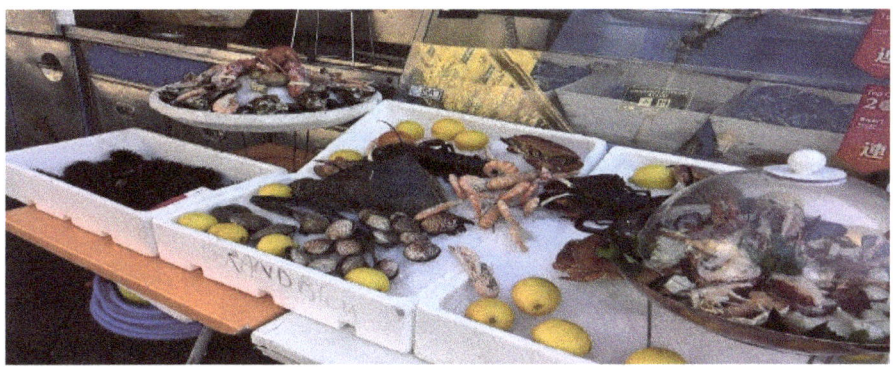

One common food allergen is shellfish. Shellfish such as crab and lobster are commonly associated with reactions amongst people. Generally this kind of reaction is seen in adulthood. There are two types of shellfish categories: crustaceans and molluscs. Crustaceans are prawns, shrimp, crab, crayfish and lobster. Molluscs are muscles, octopus, oysters, clams, snails and squid. People can either react to one singular shellfish or the group as a whole. There are many symptoms such as swelling of the lips, tongue or throat, nausea, rashes, abdominal pain and wheezing. In worst cases anaphylaxis can occur, which is a serious life-threatening condition.

Lactose intolerance is another commonly seen condition. Some people develop lactose intolerance later in life. Lactose is present in milk and dairy products and is a combination of glucose and galactose. The body needs lactase in order to break down the lactose, however, some people do not produce enough. Where this is the case the lactose sits in the gut and is fermented by bacteria. It is this process that causes symptoms such as bloating, diarrhoea and stomach cramps. Avoiding milk products and using alternative milk such as soya, goats, almond, rice or oat is recommended. Lactose intolerance can be more commonly seen in people from African and Asian culture.

Digestive System

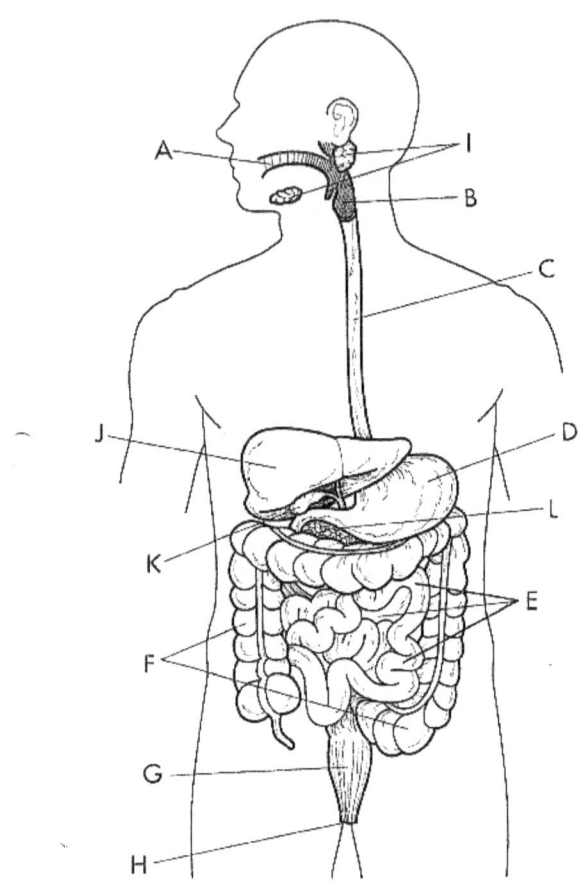

A:	B:
C:	D:
E:	F:
G:	H:
I:	J:
K:	L:

Nutrition Knowledge Quiz

1

Is water:
A: 2 hydrogen atoms and 1 oxygen atom
B: 1 hydrogen atom and 2 oxygen atoms
C: 2 hydrogen and 2 oxygen atoms

2

Where does the gallbladder lie?
A: between the liver and the pancreas
B: just below the liver
C: behind the stomach

3

What enzyme does saliva contain?
A: gastric amylase
B: salivary amylase
C: gastric Lipase

4

What is chyme?
A: a mixture of stomach acid and food
B: partially digested food
C: part of faeces

5

Refined sugar undergoes a process where:
A: sucrose is extracted from the plant
B: fructose is extracted from the plant
C: both of the above

6

Bread, Rice and Pasta are all part of the food group:
A: fats
B: carbohydrates
C: proteins

7

The immune system is triggered by:
A: an allergy
B: a food intolerance
C: both of the above

8

Which food group provides the most immediate source of energy?
A: dairy foods such as milk and cheese
B: proteins such as meat and fish
C: cereals bread and grains

9
What is the purpose of carbohydrates?
A: to help the body absorb vitamin E
B: to provide the body with energy
C: to help with digestion

10
How much of an adult's body weight is water?
A: a third
B: two thirds
C: half

Answers:
1B, 2B, 3B, 4B, 5A, 6B, 7A, 8C, 9B and 10B.

Chapter 10

Operating Biofeedback and Bioresonance Device

This section is describing how the operational functions of a biofeedback and bioresonance device work. It is describing the particular function of the Multiple Analytical Resonance System (MARS lll) as it is the one that has been used by the author. However, there are many excellent bioresonance and biofeedback devices to choose from and each of them will have different software options as well as varying operational functions. The principle of the therapy is the same and it is up to each practitioner to research and find the device that suits them best for their practice.

Described below is the operational procedure and overall basis for using a bioresonance and biofeedback device. It is purely to just give an overview to any interested party into how a bioresonance device functions from being switched on through to finishing the test procedure.

MARS III Bioresonance Device

HOW TO USE:

Make sure the computers are all turned on and running.

Turn on the bioresonance device (switch at back of machine), will take a few minutes to turn on and talk to the computer. Be patient and wait until the writing on the machine has completed its picture.

Click upon the icon 'SCOPE 4' on bottom tool bar. Again takes a few minutes to open.

Programme will open on the front page – select from the left-hand side – PATIENTS.

TO ENTER A NEW PATIENT (always check they are not existing patients first):

Select and click on the top tool bar ADD NEW PATIENTS.
Message appears – insert patient witness (hair sample/nails) – so put the patient sample in the input pot on the machine – click OK.
Machine will then scan and a message will appear – Scan Complete.
A new patient record will appear.

Complete Patient Personal Information page.
Go to the next page – additional Information on the headings tab – again complete from Patient's information. If no time of birth given by patient – add 12.00.
Next page to complete from the headings tab – Notes – add patient's medical history and reasons for the scan.
When complete – click OK at the bottom of the record, which will close record down.

Click on TEST WIZARD on left-hand margin (the patient's name will now appear as the 'Selected Patient' at the top of the screen).
Click on MAIN TEST on the right-hand margin.
Click on AUTOMATIC and using the down arrow select the test you need to perform e.g. Wheat and Gluten or Lactose and Dairy.

Results will appear on the right-hand side. Click on RESULTS and the results will be arranged in ascending order. Save Test and a message will come up wanting you to name the Test – add the Test Name and date.
Select PRINT and then REPORT and the results will appear in a Word Document.

Before saving the report:
Go to the tool bar and select Table – delete column and remove the columns marked LVL, Current Value and the blank column (one by one).
Delete Focusing and Description from the heading.
Copy the Record including Patient's name to the end of the table, paste the results into the appropriate letter.
Find the template letter in Mars III under documents – check whether a private patient or a campaign customer (Groupon/Wowcher/Living Social etc.).
Paste the results into the letter at correct spot, adding customer's name in salutation and date, your initials as a reference at the top.
Once all the tests are complete, save letter and file in appropriate folder ('results to be checked').
Delete the results form.
Complete any more tests and results the Patient requires in the same way.
Remove Patient's sample from Cup and throw away.
Go on to next patient, complete same way as above.

FIND AN EXISTING PATIENT/TO DO A NEW TEST
Click upon PATIENTS in left-hand margin.
Enter the patient's name in LAST NAME, carriage return will bring up anyone with that name.
Select the Correct Patient and left click upon their name.

Click upon SELECT at the top of records and the selected patient's name will appear at the top of the records.

UPDATE PATIENT RECORDS
If the Patient's details need to be updated/changed select PROPERTIES from top tool bar.

NEW TESTS
Click on TEST WIZARD on the left-hand margin.
The Test Wizard Page appears and you can see which tests have already been done.

Carry out any tests the patient requires in the same way as above.

NOTE – PATIENT SAMPLES ARE NOT REQUIRED FOR ANY FUTURE TESTING.
DATABASE: retains all the information for future testing, providing the information remains the same.

Chapter 11

Common Food Sensitivity and Intolerance Tests including information on how to correlate the results – Case Studies

In this chapter we describe, explain and assess the results of the food tests based on the hair sample and personal information programmed into the device.

At this stage the entire procedure of processing and entering the personal information from the health form into the bioresonance/biofeedback device, including scanning the hair sample, has been completed. All this information is logged into the computer and the hardware, the device, and has run the programme based on what the practitioner has requested.

In this section we are primarily concerned with a range of food tests but we have also interjected a couple of other tests for the student, practitioner and patient to see for interest.

Assuming that the test has already been carried out by the practitioner, the following case studies show the results that have been identified from the hair sample and have been correlated by scanning and matching the top foods for the patient/client to avoid at the present time of scanning. These foods will be either foods that the patient does not like, does not eat, have a known or unknown reaction to. Also these foods may be responsible for symptoms described on their health form (either in the short term or long term). In any event the resonance/vibrational information will be noted as a percentage by the side of a particular food that requires the patient to avoid or eliminate from the diet. A three-month period of elimination is a good idea as it gives the body time to desensitise to the particular food and/or drink. After this time it is advised to try a little of the food to see if it can be tolerated by the body. It is usually obvious whether the sensitivity has decreased as the symptoms are usually noticed once more. If the body has had a chance to cleanse or desensitise itself of a particular food, for whatever reason, it is possible and also likely that it will be tolerated after this period of elimination.

However, if the symptoms are noticed once more, then it is more likely that the food(s) is responsible for intolerance in the long term. It is advisable for the practitioner to suggest that the patient has a further test in three months to check for any changes towards the top priority foods that have been flagged up as sensitivities.

Below we will see how a food sensitivity test is interpreted, the symptoms and the results correlated to produce a plan of action for the patient.

Common Food Intolerance Tests

Examples of Types of Food Tests Shown Here

Here is a list of some of the types of food tests we have found popular and helpful to patients/clients over the years.

The Gold Standard Food Test
The first test here is the Gold Standard test that has been designed to show the practitioner a combination of three main tests that are the most popular. They consist of:
1. Standard food test showing a range of foods such as fruit, vegetables (raw and cooked), meat, fish, drinks, spices, herbs etc.
2. Dairy and Lactose.
3. Wheat and Gluten.

Each of these have a database which is used to define a much more accurate set of results as they are in a more selective list which expands on the particular type of food group.

Standard Food Test

The Standard Food Test scans a cross section of **200 food and drinks** from the database as mentioned above.

Cocoa (uncooked and chocolate bean)
Chocolate
Cereal or Grain products
Barley
Bread, wholemeal
Bread, white
Gluten
Rice
Rye
Sesame
Soya
Spelt
Pasta
Wheat
Milk
Milk (sour)
Milk
Rice milk
Yoghurt
Beer
Chocolate
Cocoa
Coffee (black)
Tea black
Tea (green)
Tea (white)
Whisky
Wine (general)
Oils, general
Olive oil
Vegetable fat
Vegetable oil
Fruit Raw
Apples
Apricots
Avocado

Bananas
Blueberries
Blackberries
Blackcurrants
Cherries
Currants (red, black etc.)
Dates
Figs
Gooseberries
Kiwis
Grapefruit
Grapes (red)
Grapes (white)
Honeydew melon
Meat
Bacon
Beef
Beef, dried
Chicken
Chicken (capon)
Duck
Egg
Egg white
Egg yolk
Goat
Goose
Ground nuts
Hazel nuts
Peanuts
Pecan nuts
Walnuts
Salmon
Smoked Salmon
Sardine
Shellfish
Shrimp
Potted Shrimps
Smoked herring, bloater
Sole
Trout (brown)
Trout (sea)
Whitefish

Cinnamon
Cumin
Curry
Ginger
Sage
Salt
Thyme
Turmeric
Vinegar (clear)
Vinegar (malt)
Yeast
Sweeteners
Confectionery, general
Honey
Maple
Molasses
Rock candy
Sugar
Beans (green)
Beans (lima)
Beans (navy)
Beets
Cabbage
Capsicum (green)
Capsicum (red)
Capsicum (yellow)
Carrots
Cauliflower – fennel
Celery
Courgettes
Mushrooms
Mustard (green)
Okra
Onion
Peas
Peas (field)
Potatoes
Garlic
Head lettuce
Olives (black)
Olives (green)
Onions

Parsley
Radish
Scarlet runner beans
Swede
Tomatoes
Watercress
Fruit Cooked
Apples
Apricots
Blueberries
Blackberries
Cherries
Cranberries
Gooseberries
Grapefruit
Peaches
Pineapples
Plums
Quince
Raisins
Raspberries

Wheat and Gluten Food Test

This test scans across all the most popular grains, example shown below:

Bread Wholemeal/ Brown	White Bread	Wheat	Gluten	Cornflakes	Cornflour/ Maize Flour	Millet
Pasta	Polenta	Porridge oats	Quinoa	Rice	Rye	Sesame
Soya	Spelt	Barley	Buckwheat	Yeast*	Noodles	Malt

Most devices will be able to have a feature that allows the practitioner to adapt, amend and add to the database. The above chart is just an example of this food group.

Dairy and Lactose Food Test

This test scans across all the most popular foods and drinks associated with dairy and lactose including some that are used as substitutes by people as they believe that some nut or rice milks may be beneficial. This is not always the case so we include them as part of our test.

Milk	Yoghurt	Rice Milk	Cream	Crème fraiche	Butter	Buttermilk
Cheese	Blue Cheese	Camembert	Cheddar	Cottage cheese	Feta	Goat's Cheese
Brie	Mozzarella	Lactose	Almond Milk	Curd	Hazelnut Milk	Paneer cheese
Soya Milk	Yoghurt Drinks	Goat's Milk				

Most devices will be able to have a feature that allows the practitioner to adapt, amend and add to the database. The above chart is just an example of this food group.

Fruit Food Test (Raw and Cooked)

This scan tests for both raw and cooked fruits

Apples	Apricots	Avocado	Banana	Bilberries	Blackberries	Blackcurrants
Blueberries	Cherries	Currants	Dates	Figs	Gooseberries	Grapefruit
Grapes (Red)	Grapes (White)	Guava	Honeydew Melon	Kiwi	Lemons	Limes
Mango	Melon	Nectarines	Oranges	Papaya	Peaches	Pears
Pink Grapefruit	Plums, Damsons	Pomegranate	Prunes	Raisins	Raspberries	Satsumas
Strawberries	Sultanas	Water Melons				

Alcohol Test

This scans across the most popular alcohols but can be added to or amended to suit cultural differences or tastes.

Beer	Bitter	Brandy	Champagne	Cider	Cognac	Gin
Guinness	Lager	Port	Red Wine	Rosé Wine	Rum	Sambuca
Schnapps	Sherry	Vodka	Whiskey	White Rum	White Wine	

Case Studies

The following case studies are examples of results that can be produced by a biofeedback/bioresonance device; please understand that all devices will produce a different appearance in columns, rates, and levels. These features are just design features and do not affect the actual results of a test. It is up to each student to become familiar with the device they have chosen. There is normally product training offered by the manufacturers with each device purchased.

Important Information

The case study below shows the first test which the biofeedback/bioresonance device has identified. This is how the device used here is programmed to deliver the results. From this first draft the practitioner will need to edit the results so that it is in a format that the patient can easily understand. The column with the level and the current value in colour can be deleted as it is not useful for the patient. The column with the percentages, however, is best put into a numerical order with the highest percentage at the top which represents the priority foods identified as sensitive at the moment.

Each biofeedback/bioresonance device will present a different visual, but if the database in that device includes a good variety of foods it will identify a list of foods to avoid, which is the most important information the patient/client will need.

Understanding and Interpreting the percentages

Please note: If the practitioner is using the Bruce Copen device and a result of 100% and a result of 0% are indicated they are to be both understood as extreme results. (This may vary with other devices used.)

If using the Bruce Copen device the results above indicate a high resonance identifying priorities and must be understood as such. This is based on experience of twenty years of practice. The principles of interpreting these results are to understand them, as any extreme result must be acknowledged. This means that the practitioner looks at the results and amends the chart to show a clearer picture for their patient. This requires skill, knowledge and experience.

See the case study results below this one to compare the differences of before and after.

All Case Studies are shown here with anonymous names and addresses to protect identities. However, the symptoms, height/weight/occupation and results are listed to help the practitioners correlate the data and therefore learn how to understand and interpret the results. However, they are based on actual people who have presented with symptoms and have chosen to have a food test to determine which foods to leave out of their diet.

Please remember that not all health symptoms are food related.

Case Studies

The following case studies are examples of food sensitivity tests.

Gold Standard Food test comprising of three separate food tests as follows:

> This food test contains three separate food tests to give a much more accurate assessment of food groups. The reason for this is that I have found it more finely tuned when looked at in a slightly more concentrated way and can give much clearer results. This is why there are a variety of tests to choose from. As a practitioner you will find this very useful to tailor your tests to your needs and of course your patient's needs and symptoms.

Case Study 1.
Gold Standard Test

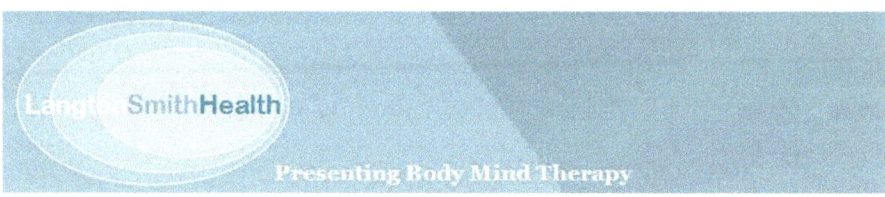

Health Form

Title MS		First Name A		Last Name Individual		
Full Address	1 ROAD					
UK				Postcode	ANY CODE 123	
Phone	0123456			Mobile	9876543	
Email	A.INDIVIDUAL@EMAIL.CO.UK					
Date of Birth	01/01/1970	Place of Birth including town and country		ANY TOWN, ENGLAND		
Male/Female	F	Height	5' 3"		Weight	9 stone
Occupation	LIBRARIAN		GP Name/Address If known		SURGERY, ANY TOWN	

Brief medical history (if any)
BLOATING /WEIGHT FLUCTUATION

List of Symptoms (if any)
BLOATING, LOW MOOD.

Specify test purchased: i.e. Wheat. Dairy. Standard Food. Full Health etc:
GOLD STANDARD FOOD TEST

Signed ....XXXXXX.....................................
Date ...01/01/2017..............................

REMEMBER TO ENCLOSE A SMALL SAMPLE OF HAIR OR FINGERNAILS (APPROX. 10 HAIRS 1 CM OR ¼ INCH LENGTH MINIMUM)
Please send the completed form and hair sample to:
Langton Smith Health

Comments

The health form above indicates that this patient is a female; she is nine stone and is experiencing symptoms of bloating, weight fluctuation and low mood. She has requested a Gold Standard Food test which looks at all three tests. A standard food test, wheat/gluten test and a dairy/lactose test.

The food test below shows the results in their raw format as they appear immediately after running the test.

Patient Name   MS. A INDIVIDUAL (0000)
Session Name   GOLD STANDARD FOOD TEST JANUARY 2016
Session Date
Focusing
Description

Rate	Lvl	Current Value	
Diet and Nutrition -> Alcohol -> Brandy	12		33
Diet and Nutrition -> Alcohol -> Cider	11		76
Diet and Nutrition -> Alcohol -> Rosé	4		46
Diet and Nutrition -> Alcohol -> Sherry	12		96
Diet and Nutrition -> Alcohol -> Sparkling Wine	3		100
Diet and Nutrition -> Cereal or Grain Products -> Noodles	4		52
Diet and Nutrition -> chocolate -> Chocolate Confectionery	10		65
Diet and Nutrition -> Dairy Products -> Feta	11		40
Diet and Nutrition -> Dairy Products -> Milk (sour)	2		27
Diet and Nutrition -> Dairy Products -> Milk (sweet)	5		57
Diet and Nutrition -> Dairy Products -> Mozzarella	1		13
Diet and Nutrition -> Drinks -> Beer	3		91
Diet and Nutrition -> Drinks -> Cocoa (with cream and sugar)	12		21
Diet and Nutrition -> Drinks -> Gin	3		74
Diet and Nutrition -> Drinks -> Ovaltine	11		42
Diet and Nutrition -> Drinks -> Tea (with cream and sugar)	2		43
Diet and Nutrition -> Fats, general -> Oils, general	9		5
Diet and Nutrition -> Fats, general -> Peppermint oil	3		36
Diet and Nutrition -> Food preparation -> Bottles	1		59
Diet and Nutrition -> Fruit (cooked) -> Bilberries	1		21
Diet and Nutrition -> Fruit (cooked) -> Cranberries	4		72
Diet and Nutrition -> Fruit (cooked) -> Pineapples	1		78
Diet and Nutrition -> Fruit (cooked) -> Plums	4		29
Diet and Nutrition -> Fruit (Raw) -> Blackcurrants	1		6
Diet and Nutrition -> Fruit (Raw) -> Mango	8		39
Diet and Nutrition -> Meat -> Duck, domestic	8		44
Diet and Nutrition -> Metabolism -> Enzymes	10		44
Diet and Nutrition -> Nuts -> Safflower	1		55
Diet and Nutrition -> Sea food/Fish -> Crayfish	11		81
Diet and Nutrition -> Sea food/Fish -> Eel	12		36
Diet and Nutrition -> Sea food/Fish -> Fish (general, fresh water)	1		36
Diet and Nutrition -> Sea food/Fish -> Herring	6		5
Diet and Nutrition -> Sea food/Fish -> Mackerel	10		20
Diet and Nutrition -> Sea food/Fish -> Plaice	5		99
Diet and Nutrition -> Spices -> Paprika	10		23

Diet and Nutrition -> Spices -> Rosemary	9		86
Diet and Nutrition -> Spices -> Sage	3		33
Diet and Nutrition -> Spices -> Salt	4		61
Diet and Nutrition -> Spices -> Turmeric	1		3
Diet and Nutrition -> Spices -> Yeast	3		40
Diet and Nutrition -> Vegetables (cooked) -> Aubergine	9		9
Diet and Nutrition -> Vegetables (cooked) -> Beans (green)	4		65
Diet and Nutrition -> Vegetables (cooked) -> Beans, navy	7		47
Diet and Nutrition -> Vegetables (cooked) -> Butternut squash	10		20
Diet and Nutrition -> Vegetables (cooked) -> Capsicum (red)	5		98
Diet and Nutrition -> Vegetables (cooked) -> Chard	6		36
Diet and Nutrition -> Vegetables (cooked) -> Potatoes	12		43
Diet and Nutrition -> Vegetables (raw) -> Bamboo Shoots	11		0
Diet and Nutrition -> Vegetables (raw) -> Head lettuce	7		36
Diet and Nutrition -> Vegetables (raw) -> Radish	6		59

The results require being put into order and in a format that the patient/client will understand.

Once the results have been edited to make more sense so that the patient is able to understand what the results mean, they are ready to be placed into a letter template of the practitioner's choosing. As can be seen by these results, in putting the 100% and 0% together, the chart looks easier to comprehend. Taking away the blue lines or any other unnecessary columns is important for the patient to understand their results. We are then left with a chart that can be understood and therefore commented on so that the patient has a clear understanding of which foods to avoid.

Results after formatting into order

Rate	
Diet and Nutrition -> Alcohol -> Sparkling Wine	100
Diet and Nutrition -> Vegetables (raw) -> Bamboo Shoots	100
Diet and Nutrition -> Sea food/Fish -> Plaice	99
Diet and Nutrition -> Vegetables (cooked) -> Capsicum (red)	98
Diet and Nutrition -> Alcohol -> Sherry	96
Diet and Nutrition -> Drinks -> Beer	91
Diet and Nutrition -> Spices -> Rosemary	86
Diet and Nutrition -> Sea food/Fish -> Crayfish	81
Diet and Nutrition -> Fruit (cooked) -> Pineapples	78
Diet and Nutrition -> Alcohol -> Cider	76
Diet and Nutrition -> Drinks -> Gin	74
Diet and Nutrition -> Fruit (cooked) -> Cranberries	72
Diet and Nutrition -> chocolate -> Chocolate Confectionery	65
Diet and Nutrition -> Vegetables (cooked) -> Beans (green)	65
Diet and Nutrition -> Spices -> Salt	61
Diet and Nutrition -> Vegetables (raw) -> Radish	59

Diet and Nutrition -> Dairy Products -> Milk	57
Diet and Nutrition -> Nuts -> Safflower	55
Diet and Nutrition -> Cereal or Grain Products -> Noodles	52
Diet and Nutrition -> Vegetables (cooked) -> Beans	47
Diet and Nutrition -> Alcohol -> Rose Wine	46
Diet and Nutrition -> Meat -> Duck	44
Diet and Nutrition -> Metabolism -> Enzymes	44
Diet and Nutrition -> Drinks -> Tea	43
Diet and Nutrition -> Vegetables (cooked) -> Potatoes	43
Diet and Nutrition -> Drinks -> Ovaltine	42
Diet and Nutrition -> Dairy Products -> Feta	40
Diet and Nutrition -> Spices -> Yeast	40
Diet and Nutrition -> Fruit (Raw) -> Mango	39
Diet and Nutrition -> Fats, general -> Peppermint oil	36
Diet and Nutrition -> Sea food/Fish -> Eel	36
Diet and Nutrition -> Sea food/Fish -> Fish (general, fresh water)	36
Diet and Nutrition -> Vegetables (cooked) -> Chard	36
Diet and Nutrition -> Vegetables (raw) -> lettuce	36
Diet and Nutrition -> Alcohol -> Brandy	33
Diet and Nutrition -> Spices -> Sage	33
Diet and Nutrition -> Fruit (cooked) -> Plums	29
Diet and Nutrition -> Dairy Products -> Milk (sour)	27
Diet and Nutrition -> Spices -> Paprika	23
Diet and Nutrition -> Drinks -> Cocoa	21
Diet and Nutrition -> Fruit (cooked) -> Blueberries	21
Diet and Nutrition -> Sea food/Fish -> Mackerel	20
Diet and Nutrition -> Vegetables (cooked) -> Butternut squash	20
Diet and Nutrition -> Dairy Products -> Mozzarella	13
Diet and Nutrition -> Vegetables (cooked) -> Aubergine	9
Diet and Nutrition -> Fruit (Raw) -> Blackcurrants	6
Diet and Nutrition -> Fats, general -> Oils, general	5
Diet and Nutrition -> Sea food/Fish -> Herring	5
Diet and Nutrition -> Spices -> Tumeric	3

Dairy Test Results

Patient Name   MS. A INDIVIDUAL (0000)
Session Name   DAIRY AND LACTOSE JANUARY 17
Session Date
Focusing
Description

Rate	Lvl	Current Value	01/01/17
Diet and Nutrition -> Dairy Products -> Brie	1		77
Diet and Nutrition -> Dairy Products -> Feta	6		44
Diet and Nutrition -> Dairy Products -> Lactose	9		0
Diet and Nutrition -> Dairy Products -> Milk	10		86
Diet and Nutrition -> Dairy Products -> Yoghurt	5		70
Diet and Nutrition -> Dairy Products -> Rice Milk	2		79
Diet and Nutrition -> Dairy Products -> Yoghurt	1		26

Results after formatting into order

Patient Name   MS. A INDIVIDUAL (0000)
Session Name   DAIRY AND LACTOSE JANUARY 17
Session Date

Rate	
Diet and Nutrition -> Dairy Products -> Lactose	100
Diet and Nutrition -> Dairy Products -> Milk	86
Diet and Nutrition -> Dairy Products -> Rice Milk	79
Diet and Nutrition -> Dairy Products -> Brie	77
Diet and Nutrition -> Dairy Products -> Yoghurt	70
Diet and Nutrition -> Dairy Products -> Feta	44

Comments

The dairy and lactose tests indicates sensitivity with lactose at 100% and a milk sensitivity at 86%. All dairy derives from milk, so if you see 'milk' then it is indicating an overall sensitivity to dairy foods. However, there are other dairy foods listed here which means that these are the top dairy foods within this group for the patient to avoid. This result also includes lactose, so this person would be best to eliminate all dairy for a while to see if this helps the symptoms. Do not forget the symptoms when correlating the results.

Wheat and Gluten Food Test

Patient Name   MS. A INDIVIDUAL (0000)
Session Name   WHEAT AND GLUTEN JANUARY 17
Session Date
Focusing
Description

Rate	Lvl	Current Value	
Diet and Nutrition -> Cereal or Grain Products -> Bread, baguette	11		0
Diet and Nutrition -> Cereal or Grain Products -> Malt	12		58
Diet and Nutrition -> Cereal or Grain Products -> Polenta	9		0
Diet and Nutrition -> Cereal or Grain Products -> Quinoa	4		67
Diet and Nutrition -> Cereal or Grain Products -> Rice	9		32
Diet and Nutrition -> Cereal or Grain Products -> Rye	1		0
Diet and Nutrition -> Cereal or Grain Products -> Soya	9		0

Results after formatting into order

Patient Name   MS. A INDIVIDUAL (0000)
Session Name   WHEAT AND GLUTEN JANUARY 17
Session Date

Rate	
Diet and Nutrition -> Cereal or Grain Products -> Bread	100
Diet and Nutrition -> Cereal or Grain Products -> Polenta	100
Diet and Nutrition -> Cereal or Grain Products -> Rye	100
Diet and Nutrition -> Cereal or Grain Products -> Soya	100
Diet and Nutrition -> Cereal or Grain Products -> Quinoa	67
Diet and Nutrition -> Cereal or Grain Products -> Malt	58
Diet and Nutrition -> Cereal or Grain Products -> Rice	32

Comments

The chart identifies bread, polenta, rye and soya as priority foods within this group for the patient to avoid. It does not indicate wheat or gluten specifically, therefore it is helpful to ask the patient what their diet includes and if they eat a lot of this, for example, a sandwich for lunch, toast for breakfast and a soya-based meal for dinner. This will give the practitioner an idea of how to help them.

Example of the final results sent to this patient:
Overall Comments for the three tests brought together below.

Results interpreted and sent to the patient.

All alcohols appear to be highly sensitive for you. Dairy intolerance is indicated, especially the dairy foods listed individually There are a number of other foods listed here; the main one is possibly yeast as it can indicate a Candida issue. I would suggest that you consider a vitamin deficiency test or a full health test at some point, as foods may not be the main cause of your symptoms. Try the above eliminations for a while and see how you feel. Yeast intolerance would mean avoiding all foods with yeast, sugars including fruits and some vegetables. Remember that carbohydrates are sugars. The other issue here is the metabolism of digestive enzymes which would indicate that you may not be processing foods well due to a low chemical/enzyme process in your metabolism. You could try a digestive enzyme or try a natural organic cider vinegar before each meal. Please come back to me if you have any questions at all.

Questions for the Practitioner to Consider: 1. How would you correlate the results of the foods listed with the symptoms presented by this patient? 2. How would you present these results to the patient? **3.** Having the symptoms in mind what is your considered opinion of the symptom specifically linked to 'low mood'? For example, is this directly connected to food?

Case Study 2.
Wheat and Gluten Food Test

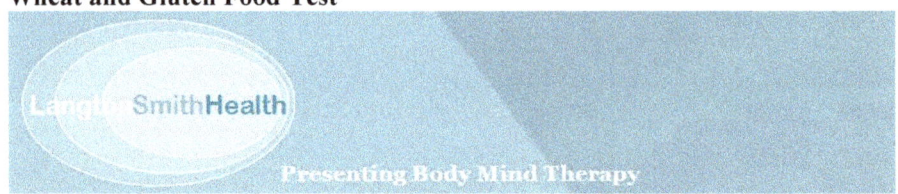

Health Form

Title MR		First Name A.B.		Last Name PERSON		
Full Address	1 STREET					
ANY PLACE						
UK				Postcode	ANY CODE 123	
Phone	0123456			Mobile	9876543	
Email	A.B.PERSON @EMAIL.CO.UK					
Date of Birth	01/01/1950		Place of Birth including town and country	ANY TOWN, ENGLAND		
Male/Female		M	Height	5' 10"	Weight	12 STONE 5LB
Occupation	ACCOUNTANT - RETIRED			GP Name/Address If known	SURGERY, ANY TOWN	

Brief medical history (if any)
DISCOMFORT AFTER EATING BREAD

List of Symptoms (if any)
DISCOMFORT AFTER EATING BREAD

Specify test purchased: i.e: Wheat. Dairy. Standard Food. Full Health etc.
WHEAT AND GLUTEN TEST

Signed ....XXXXXX......................
Date ...01/01/2017...........................

REMEMBER TO ENCLOSE A SMALL SAMPLE OF HAIR OR FINGERNAILS (APPROX. 10 HAIRS 1 CM OR ¼ INCH LENGTH MINIMUM)
Please send the completed form and hair sample to:
Langton Smith Health

Patient Name   A.B. PERSON (0000)
Session Name   WHEAT AND GLUTEN TEST JANUARY 2017
Session Date
Focusing
Description

Rate	Lvl	Current Value	
Diet and Nutrition -> Cereal or Grain Products -> Bread, baguette	6		85
Diet and Nutrition -> Cereal or Grain Products -> Bread, white bread	1		2
Diet and Nutrition -> Cereal or Grain Products -> Bread, wholemeal & Brown	2		50
Diet and Nutrition -> Cereal or Grain Products -> Millet	5		22
Diet and Nutrition -> Cereal or Grain Products -> Pasta	2		72
Diet and Nutrition -> Cereal or Grain Products -> Wheat	12		100
Diet and Nutrition -> Cereal or Grain Products -> Wheat, ground	7		2

The test results show a range of different types of bread and wheat. Looking at the symptoms for this patient it would make sense that the bloating and discomfort after eating bread is justified. There is little point in sending a set of results with a list of breads and wheat so it is best to edit the lower figures and stick to the priorities here, which are 'wheat' and 'bread'. See below how the chart has been edited to produce a final set of results with the comments for the patient.

AFTER

Patient Name   A.B. PERSON (0000)
Session Name   WHEAT AND GLUTEN TEST JANUARY 2017
Session Date
Focusing
Description

Rate	01/01/17
Diet and Nutrition -> Cereal or Grain Products -> Wheat	100
Diet and Nutrition -> Cereal or Grain Products -> Bread	85
Diet and Nutrition -> Cereal or Grain Products -> Pasta	72
Diet and Nutrition -> Cereal or Grain Products -> Millet	22

Comments

The table above shows wheat, bread and pasta to be the main foods to avoid or certainly cut back on. See if this helps with the bloating. Wheat intolerance is confirmed here. Eliminate for six months and then re-test or see how you feel without this in your diet.

Questions for the Practitioner to Consider:
1. How would you correlate the results of the foods listed with the symptoms presented by this patient?
2. How would you present these results to the patient?
3. Having the symptoms in mind what is your considered opinion of the symptom specifically linked 'discomfort after eating bread'?
4. Would age have anything to do with processing and breaking down certain foods?

Case Study 3.
Dairy and Lactose Test

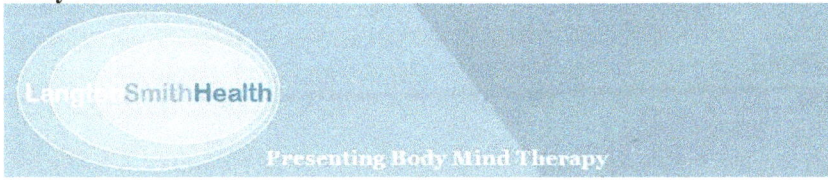

Health Form

Title MSTR		First Name O		Last Name PERSON		
Full Address	1 CRESCENT					
ANY PLACE UK				Postcode	ANY CODE 123	
Phone	0123456			Mobile	9876543	
Email	HIS.MOTHER@EMAIL.CO.UK					
Date of Birth	01/10/2011		Place of Birth including town and country		ANY TOWN, ENGLAND	
Male/Female	M	Height	4' 01"		Weight	5 STONE 4 LB
Occupation	SCHOOL STUDENT		GP Name/Address If known		SURGERY, ANY TOWN	

Brief medical history (if any)

UNSETTLED, IN PAIN

List of Symptoms (if any)

UNSETTLED, IN PAIN

Specify test purchased: i.e. Wheat. Dairy. Standard Food. Full Health etc.

DAIRY AND LACTOSE TEST

Signed ....XXXXXX.............................
Date .....01/01/2017.............................

REMEMBER TO ENCLOSE A SMALL SAMPLE OF HAIR OR FINGERNAILS (APPROX 10 HAIRS 1 CM OR ¼ INCH LENGTH MINIMUM)
Please send the completed form and hair sample to:
Langton Smith Health,

This patient is a child; pain is usually indicative of other issues, not only food. However, some foods can cause indigestion which can be painful. Please see the final chart which displays the list of foods in order of priority sensitivity. I would always refer a child back to a GP for further investigation even when finding a high sensitivity to dairy (in this case).

BEFORE

Patient Name	MSTR O. PERSON (0000)
Session Name	DAIRY AND LACTOSE TEST JANUARY 2017
Session Date
Focusing
Description

Rate	Lvl	Current Value	01/01/17
Diet and Nutrition -> Dairy Products -> Milk	12		100
Diet and Nutrition -> Dairy Products -> rice milk	10		49
Diet and Nutrition -> Dairy Products -> cottage cheese	1		76
Diet and Nutrition -> Dairy Products -> Yoghurt Drinks	2		82
Diet and Nutrition -> Dairy Products -> Hazelnut milk	10		0

AFTER

Patient Name	MSTR O. PERSON (0000)
Session Name	DAIRY AND LACTOSE TEST JANUARY 2017
Session Date	01/01/2017 01:00:00
Focusing
Description

Rate	01/01/17
Diet and Nutrition -> Dairy Products -> Milk	100
Diet and Nutrition -> Dairy Products -> Hazelnut milk	100
Diet and Nutrition -> Dairy Products -> Yoghurt Drinks	82
Diet and Nutrition -> Dairy Products -> cottage cheese	76
Diet and Nutrition -> Dairy Products -> rice milk	49

Comments

All dairy needs to be avoided for a while but even substitutes such as nut milks and rice milk are not helpful at the moment. Please email me so that we can discuss these results and try to find a way forward for him.

Further Information:
Discussed with mother and recommended further investigation with GP but to try a dairy free diet for a while to see if this helped.

Questions for the Practitioner to Consider:
1. How would you correlate the results of the foods listed with the symptoms presented by this patient?
2. How would you present these results to the patient, remembering that this is a child?
3. Having the symptoms in mind what is your considered opinion of the symptom specifically linked to feeling 'unsettled and in pain'? Is this directly connected to food?
4. What would you recommend as a practitioner?

Case Study 4.
Fruit Test

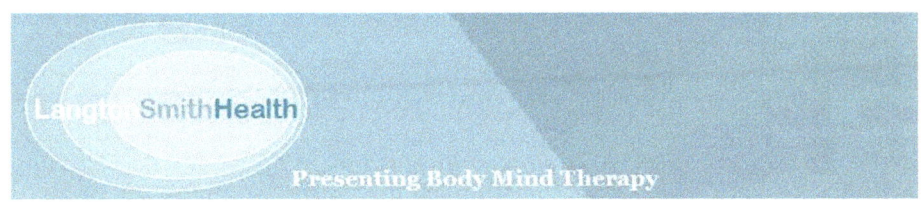

Health Form

Title MISS		First Name A.C		Last Name PERSON	
Full Address	1 STREET				
ANY PLACE					
UK				Postcode	ANY CODE 123
Phone	0123456			Mobile	9876543
Email	A.C.PERSON @EMAIL.CO.UK				
Date of Birth	01/01/2003	Place of Birth including town and country		ANY TOWN, ENGLAND	
Male/Female	F	Height	4' 8"	Weight	7 STONE
Occupation	STUDENT		GP Name/Address If known	SURGERY, ANY TOWN	

Brief medical history (if any)
MIGRAINES/HEADACHES

List of Symptoms (if any)
MIGRAINES/HEADACHES

Specify test purchased: i.e. Wheat. Dairy. Standard Food. Full Health etc.
FRUIT TEST

Signed ....XXXXXX.....................................
Date ...01/01/2017.............................

REMEMBER TO ENCLOSE A SMALL SAMPLE OF HAIR OR FINGERNAILS (APPROX. 10 HAIRS 1 CM OR ¼ INCH LENGTH MINIMUM)
Please send the completed form and hair sample to:
Langton Smith Health

BEFORE

Patient Name   MISS. A.C. PERSON (0101)
Session Name   FRUIT TEST JANUARY 2017
Session Date
Focusing
Description

Rate	Lvl	Current Value	02/06/17
Diet and Nutrition -> Fruit (cooked) -> Grapefruit	3		23
Diet and Nutrition -> Fruit (cooked) -> Lychees	3		23
Diet and Nutrition -> Fruit (cooked) -> Raisins	2		29
Diet and Nutrition -> Fruit (cooked) -> Raspberries	5		45
Diet and Nutrition -> Fruit (cooked) -> Sultanas	3		39
Diet and Nutrition -> Fruit (Raw) -> Dates	3		41
Diet and Nutrition -> Fruit (Raw) -> Gooseberries	2		75
Diet and Nutrition -> Fruit (Raw) -> Lemons	4		73
Diet and Nutrition -> Fruit (Raw) -> Oranges	3		1
Diet and Nutrition -> Fruit (Raw) -> Raisins	11		62

This is a fruit test carried out for symptoms of migraines and headaches. Notice the amount of cooked and raw raisins and sultanas mentioned here, very high in sugars, which are known to create spikes in headaches and migraines.

Patient Name MISS. A.C. PERSON (0101)
Session Name FRUIT TEST JANUARY 2017
Session Date 01/01/2017 00:00:00

Rate	01/01/17
Diet and Nutrition -> Fruit (Raw) -> Gooseberries	75
Diet and Nutrition -> Fruit (Raw) -> Lemons	73
Diet and Nutrition -> Fruit (Raw) -> Raisins	62
Diet and Nutrition -> Fruit (cooked) -> Raspberries	45
Diet and Nutrition -> Fruit (Raw) -> Dates	41
Diet and Nutrition -> Fruit (cooked) -> Sultanas	39
Diet and Nutrition -> Fruit (cooked) -> Raisins	29
Diet and Nutrition -> Fruit (cooked) -> Grapefruit	23
Diet and Nutrition -> Fruit (cooked) -> Lychees	23
Diet and Nutrition -> Fruit (Raw) -> Oranges	1

This test indicates a need to avoid all types of foods that include raisins, lemons and gooseberries, including foods such as jams and cooked fruit. It would be worth trying this elimination diet for a while to see if it has made a difference, and if not recommend a different food test for comparison as this will only give the picture regarding fruit.

Questions for the Practitioner to Consider:
1. How would you correlate the results of the foods listed with the symptoms presented by this patient?
2. How would you present these results to the patient?
3. Having the symptoms in mind, what is your considered opinion of the symptoms specifically linked to 'migraines and headaches'? Is this directly connected to food?
4. What would you suggest to the patient's mother/father?

Reading and interpreting a set of results including the correlation of symptoms with the identified results.

Final sets of results for interpretation by the practitioner:
Case Study 5.
Alcohol Test

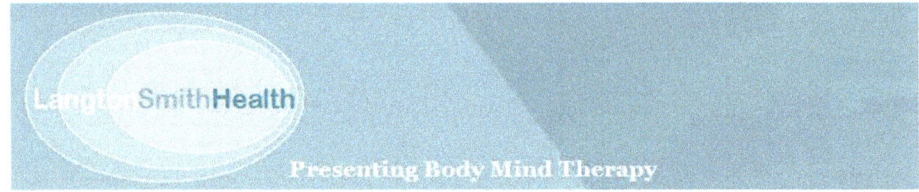

Health Form

Title MR		First Name B	Last Name SOMEONE	
Full Address	1 THE CLOSE			
ANY PLACE				
UK		Postcode	ANY CODE 123	
Phone	0123456	Mobile	9876543	
Email	B.SOMEONE@EMAIL.CO.UK			
Date of Birth	01/01/1975	Place of Birth including town and country	ANY TOWN, ENGLAND	
Male/Female	M	Height	6' 02"	Weight	12 STONE
Occupation	MECHANIC	GP Name/Address If known	SURGERY, ANY TOWN	

Brief medical history (if any)
WAKE UP AT NIGHT AFTER DRINKING

List of Symptoms (if any)
WAKE UP AT NIGHT AFTER DRINKING

Specify test purchased: i.e. Wheat. Dairy. Standard Food. Full Health etc.
ALCOHOL TEST

Signed ………XXXXXX……………………………………
Date …01/01/2017……………………………

REMEMBER TO ENCLOSE A SMALL SAMPLE OF HAIR OR FINGERNAILS (APPROX. 10 HAIRS 1 CM OR ¼ INCH LENGTH MINIMUM)
Please send the completed form and hair sample to:
Langton Smith Health

Patient Name MR B. SOMEONE (0101)
Session Name ALCOHOL TEST JANUARY 2017
Session Date 01/01/2017   00:00:00
Focusing
Description

Rate	01/01/17
Diet and Nutrition -> Alcohol -> Beer	92
Diet and Nutrition -> Alcohol -> Schnapps	88
Diet and Nutrition -> Alcohol -> Rose wine	66
Diet and Nutrition -> Alcohol -> Gin	30
Diet and Nutrition -> Alcohol -> Sherry	26

This person is waking up at night after drinking alcohol and wondering why. The alcohol test has identified beer as the main issue. It is up to the practitioner to discuss these results with the patient to see how they might be able to adapt their drinking habits to avoid waking up in the night. Other alcohols may or may not be drunk but these will show a potential sensitivity and are therefore a warning to avoid.

Questions for the Practitioner to Consider:
1. How would you correlate the results of the foods listed with the symptoms presented by this patient?
2. How would you present these results to the patient?
3. Having the symptoms in mind what is your considered opinion of the symptoms of 'waking up at night after drinking'? Is this directly connected to the alcohol?
4. How would you discuss this with the patient?

Case Study 6.
Wellness Test
Comprising of a Standard Food Test and a Vitamin Deficiency Test

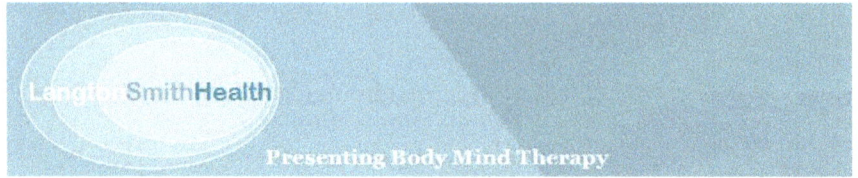

Health Form

Title MR		First Name D		Last Name SOMEBODY	
Full Address	1 THE CLOSE				
ANY PLACE					
UK			Postcode	ANY CODE 123	
Phone	0123456		Mobile	9876543	
Email	D.SOMEBODY@EMAIL.CO.UK				
Date of Birth	01/01/1982		Place of Birth including town and country	ANY TOWN, ENGLAND	
Male/Female	M	Height	5' 10"	Weight	15 STONE
Occupation	NURSERY WORKER		GP Name/Address If known	SURGERY, ANY TOWN	
Brief medical history (if any)					
OF GENERAL INTEREST					
List of Symptoms (if any)					
OF GENERAL INTEREST					
Specify test purchased: i.e. Wheat. Dairy. Standard Food. Full Health etc.					
WELLNESS FOOD AND VITAMIN TEST					

Signed ....XXXXXX.....................................
Date ...01/01/2017.............................

REMEMBER TO ENCLOSE A SMALL SAMPLE OF HAIR OR FINGERNAILS (APPROX 10 HAIRS 1 CM OR ¼ INCH LENGTH MINIMUM)
Please send the completed form and hair sample to:
Langton Smith Health

Results

Patient Name: MR D. SOMEBODY (0101)
Session Name: WELLNESS FOOD TEST JANUARY 2017
Session Date: 01/01/2017   00:00:00

Rate	07/03/16
Diet and Nutrition -> Cereal or Grain Products -> Millet	100
Diet and Nutrition -> Fruit (Raw) -> Apples	100
Diet and Nutrition -> Vegetables (cooked) -> Shallot	98
Diet and Nutrition -> Drinks -> Champagne	86
Diet and Nutrition -> Sweeteners -> White sugar	86
Diet and Nutrition -> Spices -> Vinegar (malt)	85
Diet and Nutrition -> Cereal or Grain Products -> Wheat	77
Diet and Nutrition -> Nuts -> Coconut	74
Diet and Nutrition -> Fruit (Raw) -> Dates	67
Diet and Nutrition -> Cereal or Grain Products -> Noodles	56
Diet and Nutrition -> Cereal or Grain Products -> Barley	55
Diet and Nutrition -> Drinks -> Redbush Tea	48
Diet and Nutrition -> Metabolism -> Glucose	46
Diet and Nutrition -> Dairy Products -> Yoghurt Drinks	45
Diet and Nutrition -> Alcohol -> Schnapps	44
Diet and Nutrition -> Alcohol -> Whisky	44
Diet and Nutrition -> Meat -> Roe-deer	44
Diet and Nutrition -> Cereal or Grain Products -> Porridge oats	43
Diet and Nutrition -> Dairy Products -> Almond Milk	42
Diet and Nutrition -> Vegetables (raw) -> Tomatoes	42
Diet and Nutrition -> Sea food/Fish -> Lobster	35
Diet and Nutrition -> Fruit (cooked) -> Currants	34
Diet and Nutrition -> Meat -> Lamb	31
Diet and Nutrition -> Vegetables (raw) -> Brussels sprouts	27
Diet and Nutrition -> Cereal or Grain Products -> Gluten	15
Diet and Nutrition -> Vegetables (raw) -> Olives (green)	15
Diet and Nutrition -> Sea food/Fish -> Catfish	7
Diet and Nutrition -> Meat -> Beef	5
Diet and Nutrition -> Spices -> Oregano	1

Comments

The Wellness test looks at the overall nutritional health of the patient, the foods to avoid and the vitamins required for general health and wellness.

The first chart indicates the top foods to avoid here, which include millet, apples, shallot, champagne, sugars, wheat and a few other priority foods. Gluten is listed but at a low 15% so perhaps this needs to be reduced from the diet. However, wheat-free food is best but as there are no symptoms listed it is difficult for the practitioner to know how to respond to this set of results. General interest is sometimes listed but most people have symptoms therefore this is unusual. Always best to ask the patient for symptoms so that there is an element of sense made to these results.

However, the patient does weigh 15 stone so it is important to understand what these foods mean. The sugar element and then looking down at the chart to see glucose also listed may well indicate early signs of diabetes type 2, which can often be controlled by diet.

Patient Name   MR D. SOMEBODY (0101)
Session Name   WELLNESS VITAMIN TEST JANUARY 2017
Session Date   01/01/2017   00:00:00
Focusing
Description

Rate	07/03/16
Vitamins, imbalance -> Vitamin C	73
Vitamins, imbalance -> Valine	71
Vitamins, imbalance -> Vitamin D1	40
Minerals -> Water	32
Vitamins, imbalance -> Hydroxyproline	26
Minerals -> Calcium	16

Comments

The vitamin test shows deficiency in Vitamin C and some amino acids; Vit D1 and water is indicated suggesting that this person does not drink enough and is dehydrated. Again, this represents a reasonable chart that would suggest that this person is in general good health although overweight. Whilst they have said that they are doing this test for general interest I believe that it is important to highlight the need to change the diet to a low-sugar diet to enable weight loss. I would recommend leaving certain foods out of the diet but taking a supplement of Vit C and Vit D for six months. Increase water consumption and then to see how things are.

Questions for the Practitioner to Consider:
1. How would you correlate the results of the foods listed with the symptoms presented by this patient?
2. How would you present these results to the patient?
3. Having the symptoms in mind, what is your considered opinion of the patient not declaring any symptoms and just stating that the test is for 'general interest'?
4. How would you discuss this with the patient?

Case Study 7.
Weight Loss Test

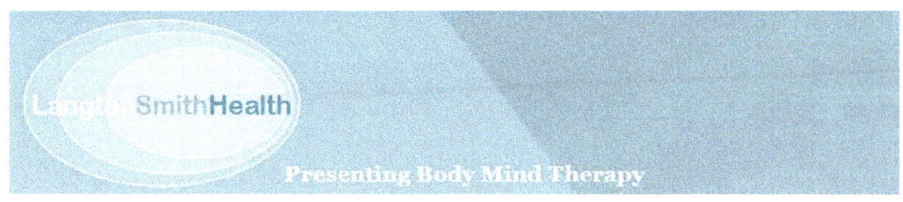

Health Form

Title		First Name		Last Name	
MRS		E		LADY	
Full Address	1 THE CROFT				
	ANY PLACE				
	UK		Postcode	ANY CODE 123	
Phone	0123456		Mobile	9876543	
Email	E.LADY@EMAIL.CO.UK				
Date of Birth	01/01/1976	Place of Birth including town and country		ANY TOWN, ENGLAND	
Male/Female	F	Height	5' 2"	Weight	11 STONE
Occupation	SECRETARY	GP Name/Address If known		SURGERY, ANY TOWN	

Brief medical history (if any)
FIND IT DIFFICULT TO LOSE WEIGHT

List of Symptoms (if any)
DRYNESS OF EYES, MOUTH

Specify test purchased: ie: Wheat. Dairy. Standard Food. Full Health etc:
WEIGHT LOSS TEST

Signed ....XXXXXX......................................
Date ...01/01/2017.............................

REMEMBER TO ENCLOSE A SMALL SAMPLE OF HAIR OR FINGERNAILS (APPROX 10 HAIRS 1 CM OR ¼ INCH LENGTH MINIMUM)
Please send the completed form and hair sample to:
Langton Smith Health

Patient Name   MRS E. LADY (0101)
Session Name   WEIGHT LOSS TEST JANUARY 2017
Session Date

Rate	02/06/17
Diet and Nutrition -> Nuts -> Sesame	100
Diet and Nutrition -> Sea food/Fish -> Bream	100
Diet and Nutrition -> Sweets- confectionary	100
Diet and Nutrition -> Vegetables (cooked) -> Potatoes	100
Diet and Nutrition -> Fruit (cooked) -> Grapefruit	99
Diet and Nutrition -> Meat -> Beef, dried (sauces and gravies)	99
Diet and Nutrition -> Meat -> Liver (lamb)	99
Diet and Nutrition -> Cereal or Grain Products -> Bread	97
Diet and Nutrition -> Drinks -> Fennel Tea	92
Diet and Nutrition -> Dairy Products -> Milk	84
Diet and Nutrition -> Vegetables (cooked) -> Maize	77
Diet and Nutrition -> Nuts -> Almond	72
Diet and Nutrition -> Fruit (Raw) -> Mango	63
Diet and Nutrition -> Fruit (cooked) -> Cherries	62
Diet and Nutrition -> Metabolism -> Acid	59
Diet and Nutrition -> Vegetables (cooked) -> Okra	58
Diet and Nutrition -> Dairy Products -> Feta	55
Diet and Nutrition -> Drinks -> Fruit Juices	46
Diet and Nutrition -> Fats, general -> Vegetable fat spreads	45
Diet and Nutrition -> Fruit (cooked) -> Oranges	43
Diet and Nutrition -> Fruit (Raw) -> Pink Grapefruit	43
Diet and Nutrition -> Vegetables (raw) -> Olives (black)	41
Diet and Nutrition -> Vegetables (raw) -> Cabbage	39
Diet and Nutrition -> Fruit (Raw) -> Grapes (white)	38
Diet and Nutrition -> chocolate -> Chocolate Confectionery	33
Diet and Nutrition -> Sea food/Fish -> Mackerel	32
Diet and Nutrition -> Vegetables (raw) -> Olives (green)	32
Diet and Nutrition -> Sea food/Fish -> Halibut	30
Diet and Nutrition -> Dairy Products -> Curd (cottage cheese)	29
Diet and Nutrition -> Dairy Products -> Soya Milk	27
Diet and Nutrition -> Meat -> Duck	26
Diet and Nutrition -> Cereal or Grain Products -> Porridge oats	23
Diet and Nutrition -> Drinks -> Verbena	22
Diet and Nutrition -> Cereal or Grain Products -> Millet	19
Diet and Nutrition -> Fats, general -> Cod liver oil	19
Diet and Nutrition -> Fruit (cooked) -> Banana	18
Diet and Nutrition -> Vegetables (cooked) -> Garlic	14
Diet and Nutrition -> Fruit (Raw) -> Apples	11
Diet and Nutrition -> Spices -> Celery Seed	9
Diet and Nutrition -> Drinks -> Redbush Tea	6
Diet and Nutrition -> Spices -> Nutmeg	4
Diet and Nutrition -> Vegetables (raw) -> Garlic	4

Comments

> The main food groups featured here for you to avoid to support weight loss are potatoes, bread and dairy. All the foods listed are contributory to weight gain or a slower weight loss than other foods. This list helps to identify the foods for you to avoid completely even if you think they are good for you they may not be helping you to achieve your goal. Avoid all sweets and chocolate as these are on this list and represent your top foods tested to avoid. If you try this for three months you may find that the dryness of your mouth and eyes improves but if not I would recommend that you consult your GP or consider a vitamin deficiency test.

Questions for the Practitioner to Consider:
5. How would you correlate the results of the foods listed with the symptoms presented by this patient?
6. How would you present these results to the patient?
7. Having the symptoms in mind, what is your considered opinion of these food test results and the connection to weight issues, dryness of the eyes and mouth?
8. How would you discuss this with the patient?

Case Study 8.
Standard Food Test

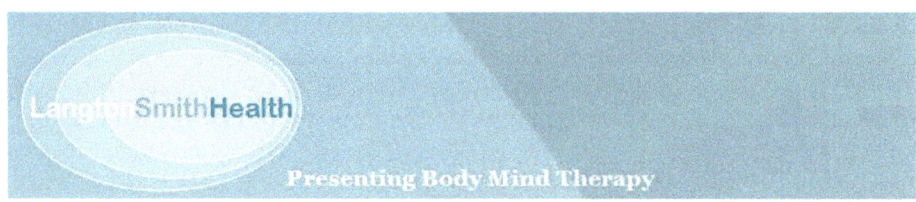

Health Form

Title MRS		First Name F.G		Last Name PERSON		
Full Address	1 THE MALL					
ANY PLACE						
UK				Postcode	ANY CODE 123	
Phone	0123456			Mobile	9876543	
Email	F.G.PERSON@EMAIL.CO.UK					
Date of Birth	01/01/1982		Place of Birth including town and country		ANY TOWN, ENGLAND	
Male/Female	F	Height		5' 7"	Weight	9 STONE 7 LB
Occupation	FITNESS TRAINER		GP Name/Address If known		SURGERY, ANY TOWN	

Brief medical history (if any)

ENERGY FLUCTUATIONS

List of Symptoms (if any)

ENERGY FLUCTUATIONS

Specify test purchased: i.e. Wheat. Dairy. Standard Food. Full Health etc.

STANDARD FOOD TEST

Signed ....XXXXXX........................
Date ...01/01/2017..............................

REMEMBER TO ENCLOSE A SMALL SAMPLE OF HAIR OR FINGERNAILS (APPROX. 10 HAIRS 1 CM OR ¼ INCH LENGTH MINIMUM)
Please send the completed form and hair sample to:
Langton Smith Health

Patient Name MRS F.G. PERSON (0000)
Session Name STANDARD FOOD TEST JANUARY 2017
Session Date 01/01/2017   00:00:00

Rate	05/12/16
Diet and Nutrition -> Alcohol -> Red Wine	0
Diet and Nutrition -> Alcohol -> Rum	46
Diet and Nutrition -> Alcohol -> Sambuca	0
Diet and Nutrition -> Dairy Products -> Brie	41
Diet and Nutrition -> Dairy Products -> Butter	0
Diet and Nutrition -> Dairy Products -> Hazelnut Milk	64
Diet and Nutrition -> Dairy Products -> Soya Milk	23
Diet and Nutrition -> Drinks -> Lager	85
Diet and Nutrition -> Drinks -> Vodka	65
Diet and Nutrition -> Fruit (cooked) -> Cherries	54
Diet and Nutrition -> Fruit (Raw) -> Dates	66
Diet and Nutrition -> Fruit (Raw) -> Nectarines	23
Diet and Nutrition -> Fruit (Raw) -> Plums, damsons	70
Diet and Nutrition -> Fruit (Raw) -> Pomegranates	88
Diet and Nutrition -> Fruit (Raw) -> Raspberries	42
Diet and Nutrition -> Meat -> Beef	68
Diet and Nutrition -> Meat -> Egg	63
Diet and Nutrition -> Nuts -> Brazil nuts	92
Diet and Nutrition -> Nuts -> Pine Nuts	17
Diet and Nutrition -> Sea food/Fish -> Mackerel	91
Diet and Nutrition -> Sea food/Fish -> Oyster	42
Diet and Nutrition -> Spices -> Cumin	52
Diet and Nutrition -> Spices -> Pepper (white)	37
Diet and Nutrition -> Spices -> Rosemary	0
Diet and Nutrition -> Sweeteners -> Maple	11
Diet and Nutrition -> Vegetables (cooked) -> Capsicum (yellow)	36
Diet and Nutrition -> Vegetables (cooked) -> Celery	39
Diet and Nutrition -> Vegetables (cooked) -> Swede	100
Diet and Nutrition -> Vegetables (raw) -> Beansprouts	26
Diet and Nutrition -> Vegetables (raw) -> Cabbage	32

AFTER

Patient Name   MRS F.G. PERSON (0000)
Session Name   STANDARD FOOD TEST JANUARY 2017
Session Date   01/01/2017   00:00:00

Rate	05/12/16
Diet and Nutrition -> Alcohol -> Red Wine	100
Diet and Nutrition -> Alcohol -> Sambuca	100
Diet and Nutrition -> Dairy Products -> Butter	100
Diet and Nutrition -> Spices -> Rosemary	100
Diet and Nutrition -> Vegetables (cooked) -> Swede	100
Diet and Nutrition -> Nuts -> Brazil nuts	92
Diet and Nutrition -> Sea food/Fish -> Mackerel	91
Diet and Nutrition -> Fruit (Raw) -> Pomegranates	88
Diet and Nutrition -> Drinks -> Lager	85
Diet and Nutrition -> Fruit (Raw) -> Plums, damsons	70
Diet and Nutrition -> Meat -> Beef	68
Diet and Nutrition -> Fruit (Raw) -> Dates	66
Diet and Nutrition -> Drinks -> Vodka	65
Diet and Nutrition -> Dairy Products -> Hazelnut Milk	64
Diet and Nutrition -> Egg	63
Diet and Nutrition -> Fruit (cooked) -> Cherries	54
Diet and Nutrition -> Spices -> Cumin	52
Diet and Nutrition -> Alcohol -> Rum	46
Diet and Nutrition -> Fruit (Raw) -> Raspberries	42
Diet and Nutrition -> Sea food/Fish -> Oyster	42
Diet and Nutrition -> Dairy Products -> Brie	41
Diet and Nutrition -> Vegetables (cooked) -> Celery	39
Diet and Nutrition -> Spices -> Pepper (white)	37
Diet and Nutrition -> Vegetables (cooked) -> Capsicum (yellow)	36
Diet and Nutrition -> Vegetables (raw) -> Cabbage	32
Diet and Nutrition -> Vegetables (raw) -> Beansprouts	26
Diet and Nutrition -> Dairy Products -> Soya Milk	23
Diet and Nutrition -> Fruit (Raw) -> Nectarines	23
Diet and Nutrition -> Nuts -> Pine Nuts	17
Diet and Nutrition -> Sweeteners -> Maple	11

Comments

The patient has mentioned about energy fluctuations and is not concerned about her weight, which is healthy. Also note that this person is a fitness trainer. The foods here show sensitivity to a variety of alcohols but the foods do not really look as though they will provide an answer to energy levels. I would either suggest a vitamin deficiency test or find out a little more about lifestyle. All these alcohols need to be avoided but maybe an alcohol-free diet for 2–3 months might help.

Questions for the Practitioner to Consider:
1. How would you correlate the results of the foods listed with the symptoms presented by this patient?
2. How would you present these results to the patient?
3. Having the symptoms in mind, what is your considered opinion of the symptoms of 'energy fluctuations'? Is this directly connected to any of the foods/drinks highlighted on the results?
4. How would you discuss this with the patient?
5. If you do not feel that this food test has provided a full picture to assist with the patient's symptoms, what would you suggest?

Case Study 9.
Wheat and Gluten Test

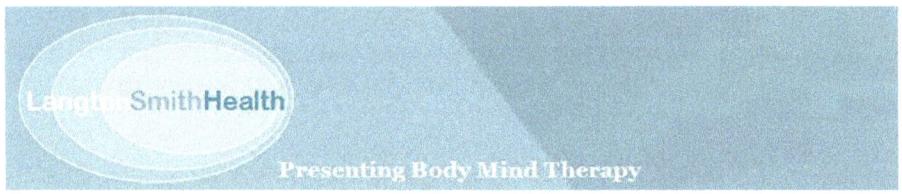

Health Form

Title MISS		First Name A		Last Name BC	
Full Address	1 THE STREET				
ANY PLACE					
UK			Postcode	ANY CODE 123	
Phone	0123456		Mobile	9876543	
Email	A.BC@EMAIL.CO.UK				
Date of Birth	01/01/1978		Place of Birth including town and country	ANY TOWN, ENGLAND	
Male/Female	F		Height	5' 3"	Weight	9 STONE
Occupation	ADMINISTRATOR		GP Name/ Address If known	SURGERY, ANY TOWN	

Brief medical history (if any)

STOMACH ACHE

List of Symptoms (if any)

STOMACH ACHE

Specify test purchased: i.e. Wheat. Dairy. Standard Food. Full Health etc.

WHEAT AND GLUTEN TEST

Signed ………XXXXXX…………………………………
Date …01/01/2017……………………………

REMEMBER TO ENCLOSE A SMALL SAMPLE OF HAIR OR FINGERNAILS (APPROX. 10 HAIRS 1 CM OR ¼ INCH LENGTH MINIMUM)
Please send the completed form and hair sample to:
Langton Smith Health

Patient Name   MS A. BC (0000)
Session Name   WHEAT AND GLUTEN TEST JANUARY 17
Session Date   01/01/2017   00:00:00

Rate	13/05/17
Diet and Nutrition -> Cereal or Grain Products -> Cornflakes	99
Diet and Nutrition -> Cereal or Grain Products -> Maize flour	97
Diet and Nutrition -> Cereal or Grain Products -> Noodles	94
Diet and Nutrition -> Cereal or Grain Products -> Rye	77
Diet and Nutrition -> Cereal or Grain Products -> Malt	47
Diet and Nutrition -> Cereal or Grain Products -> Porridge oats	24
Diet and Nutrition -> Cereal or Grain Products -> Barley	17

Comments

Avoid all foods containing corn/maize as well as the other foods listed above as they are your top priority foods indicated as sensitive for you. There may be other foods involved with the symptoms you have listed so perhaps consider a full food test at some point in the future. However, these results do not indicate wheat and gluten sensitivity. I suggest that you either consider a full food test or consult with your GP regarding your stomach ache. The wheat and gluten test only covers the list of foods connected to grains.

Questions for the Practitioner to Consider:
1. How would you correlate the results of the foods listed with the symptoms presented by this patient?
2. How would you present these results to the patient?
3. Having the symptoms of the patient's stomach ache in mind, what is your considered opinion after seeing the results which do not offer a conclusive wheat and gluten sensitivity?
4. How would you discuss this with the patient?

Case Study 10.
Vitamin Test

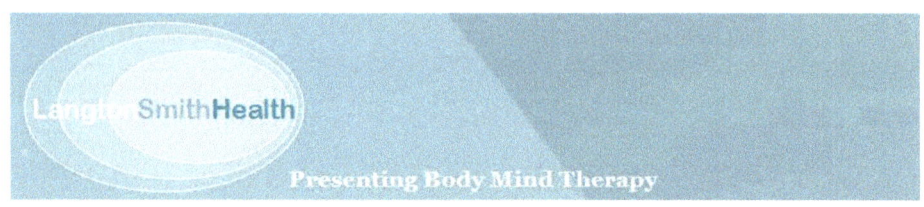

Health Form

Title		First Name		Last Name	
MRS		A		PERSON	
Full Address	1 AVENUE				
ANY PLACE					
UK				Postcode	ANY CODE 123
Phone		0123456		Mobile	9876543
Email		A.PERSON@EMAIL.CO.UK			
Date of Birth		01/01/1966		Place of Birth including town and country	ANY TOWN, ENGLAND
Male/Female		F	Height	5' 7"	Weight	13 STONE
Occupation		MANAGER		GP Name/Address If known	SURGERY, ANY TOWN

Brief medical history (if any)
TIREDNESS /FATIGUE

List of Symptoms (if any)
FATIGUE, TROUBLE CONCENTRATING.

Specify test purchased: ie: Wheat. Dairy. Standard Food. Full Health etc:
VITAMIN TEST

Signed ………XXXXXX……………………………
Date …01/01/2017……………………

REMEMBER TO ENCLOSE A SMALL SAMPLE OF HAIR OR FINGERNAILS (APPROX. 10 HAIRS 1 CM OR ¼ INCH LENGTH MINIMUM)
Please send the completed form and hair sample to:
Langton Smith Health

Patient Name   A. PERSON (0101)
Session Name   VITAMIN TEST JANUARY 2017
Session Date   01/07/2017 10:30:56

Rate	01/01/17
Minerals -> Cadmium	100
Vitamins, imbalance -> L-Carnitine	84
Vitamins, imbalance -> Co Q 10	64
Vitamins, imbalance -> leucine	64
Vitamins, imbalance -> Histidine	28
Minerals -> Zinc	10

Comments

Cadmium is a toxin that is in fertilisers, cigarettes etc., and it is shown here as a sensitivity, which is either due to a high sensitivity to certain items that contain this or something that this patient is doing to attract this toxin such as smoking. However, if the liver is overloaded due to a diet of high carbohydrates/sugars then a sensitivity towards chemicals and metals is noticed.

I would recommend a full food test (standard) to see what this patient might benefit from eliminating from their diet to see if this helps energy levels and fatigue. This patient is overweight, which may well contribute towards tiredness and fatigue. More investigation would be required here. However, starting the patient off with a general broad spectrum amino acid complex may help or the super food Spirulina.

However, the energy levels may be helped by trying the amino acid L Carnitine, which is thought to help improve energy; Co Q 10 is another vitamin for cellular energy and as there are two other amino acids mentioned it may well be helpful to consider an amino acid complex. This is explained in more detail in our next course.

Questions for the Practitioner to Consider:
1. How would you correlate the results of the foods listed with the symptoms presented by this patient?
2. How would you present these results to the patient?
3. Having patients' symptoms in mind, 'tiredness, fatigue, difficulty in concentrating', what would you suggest that may help the patient based on the vitamin deficiency test results?
4. How would you discuss this with the patient?
5. Would you consider anything else that might help the patient with her symptoms?

Chapter 12

Creating a template letter to send results to a patient/client

The results that have been identified by the bioresonance/biofeedback device need to now be placed into a letter that includes some information about the testing methods and also some information with regard to food sensitivities and food intolerances. Below are some letter templates that will give the practitioner an idea of how to format a template to help with their explanation and meanings of the results. Each practitioner will have their own personal method of tailoring their work to suit their particular speciality.

Example of Wheat and Gluten and/or Dairy Lactose Letter Template:

Dear
Thank you for choosing to take a Gluten/Wheat Sensitivity Test with Langton Smith Health.

Food sensitivity may be a temporary issue that requires a short period of time to desensitise the body to certain foods. We have found that three months is a good period of time to limit the specified foods and allow the body to cleanse itself of those foods that have caused symptoms. These may include bloating, stomach cramps, acidity, IBS etc.

If you are doing this for curiosity then it might help to try eliminating the foods shown in your top 2 personal results below.

Some foods may be shown that you do not eat. This is because the medical scanner will identify any potential sensitivity that may occur whether eaten or not. Please remember that not all symptoms are food related.

Comments Below
The higher the percentage number means the higher the sensitivity
The top lists are your priority foods based on the tables 1 and 2 of foods tested at the end of this report.

RESULTS INSERTED HERE

Understanding your food sensitivity results:

70–100 = High sensitivity: eliminate or reduce these foods as much as possible
40–70 = Medium sensitivity: reduce or limit these foods in your diet
1–40 = Low Sensitivity: eat these foods sensibly (in moderation)

Avoid any of the foods listed above that are applicable to your diet for approximately three months so that you can monitor any changes to your health/digestion. As we do not have information regarding your current diet or lifestyle, it might be interesting for you to follow the recommendations above to see if it makes a difference to your overall health.

Common Food Sensitivities Explained

Bread: When bread is indicated with a *medium or high* figure this means it needs to be avoided, even if it is wheat or gluten free. This is often due to its consistency, which can be difficult for some people to digest.

Yeast: When yeast is indicated with a *medium or high* figure, this normally means to avoid bread and any food that contains yeast, including foods such as fruit/juices, alcohol (beers, lagers), sweets and refined sugars, as these foods act as triggers for yeast growth. It may also be helpful to take a good probiotic capsule for three months to help stabilise the gut flora and support the immune system.

Gluten: When gluten is indicated with a *medium or high* figure, it is recommended to avoid all grains that contain gluten for approximately three months. These include wheat, barley, rye, semolina, spelt and couscous. These are found in foods such as bread (including breadcrumbs), rolls, chapattis, biscuits, crackers, cakes, pastries, pizza, pasta, gravies and sauces etc. Below are examples of some of the foods that contain wheat and gluten.

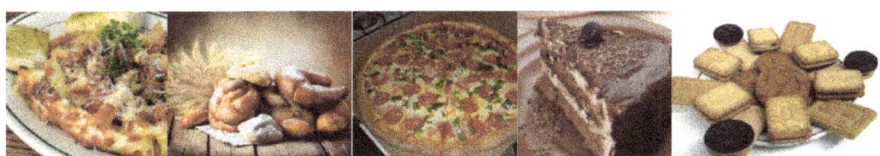

Suggested replacement foods:
Corn, rice, rice flour, amaranth, buckwheat, millet, teff, quinoa, sorghum, soya flour, potato starch, modified starch, potato flour, gram flour, polenta (cornmeal), sago, tapioca, cassava.

We do not recommend eating gluten-free foods as they tend to be expensive and some are genetically modified to make them gluten free, however this is your decision to make.

Dairy: When milk is indicated with a *medium or high* figure, it is recommended to avoid *all* dairy. This is because all dairy derives from milk. Below are examples of foods that contain dairy.

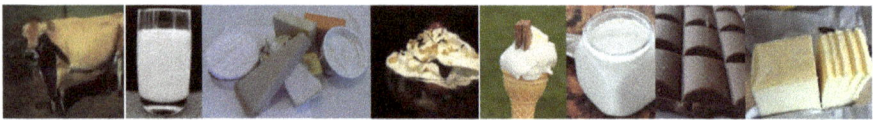

Suggested replacement foods

Dairy free:
As all dairy originates from a cow, it is advised to adapt your diet to other types of dairy-free or alternatives such as soy, nut milks, rice milks, goat and sheep products.

How to Understand your Results
There are two tables below that represent all the Dairy and Wheat foods that are tested. From this table *only the priority foods* are indicated on your personal results in percentage terms above.

Your personal test results indicate the main foods that are showing as a sensitivity/or potential sensitivity to you at the moment.

Table 1. Lactose/Dairy Foods Tested

Milk	Yoghurt	Rice Milk	Cream	Crème fraiche	Butter	Buttermilk
Cheese	Blue Cheese	Camembert	Cheddar	Cottage cheese	Feta	Goat's cheese
Brie	Mozzarella	Lactose	Almond Milk	Curd	Hazelnut Milk	Paneer cheese
Soya Milk	Yoghurt Drinks	Goat's Milk				

Table 2. Gluten/Wheat Foods Tested

Bread wholemeal/ brown	White Bread	Wheat	Gluten	Cornflakes	Cornflour/ Maize Flour	Millet
Pasta	Polenta	Porridge oats	Quinoa	Rice	Rye	Sesame
Soya	Spelt	Barley	Buckwheat	Yeast*	Noodles	Malt

Symptoms

Please have in mind that this test is only scanning for dairy and wheat foods and is *not* a full food test. This means that other foods may be sensitive for you and so this test may not provide the entire solution to your health symptoms. We suggest that you start with eliminating the foods listed here, if appropriate for you, and then contact us again if you need to discuss your health symptoms in more detail.

About our Food tests:
Our Food Tests are based on bioresonance therapy, a complementary medical approach to health. All tests are conducted using a medical scanning device which has an EU medical classification and is covered by the European ISO standard regulations. Hair samples are used to identify a variety of health-related issues and each test is tailored to the individual.

Heading up the team is Julie Langton Smith MSc, bioresonance nutritional practitioner and naturopath who oversees each food test result letter before it is sent. All our tests are personalised to each individual and the offer to discuss your test results is made clear so that if there is anything at all that you need clarification on, please do not hesitate to contact us.

Please note that there may be foods listed that you do not like and would not eat but this test indicates a potential sensitivity that these foods are best avoided. If you know that you already have a problem with a specific food type and have not eaten them for a while it is quite normal for these foods not to show up as they will not be showing a resonance in the body.

Always contact us if you are unsure of your results, we are very happy to explain them to you.

We wish you the very best of health.
Kind regards

Julie Langton Smith MSc
MGHRC, MFHT, MNCS, PSA
Bioresonance Nutritional Practitioner and Psychotherapist
www.langtonsmithhealth.com/

Professional Disclaimer: Please remember that this is complementary medicine and does not form part of any conventional medical process. I have been practising for many years as a nutritional healthcare practitioner specialising in bioresonance therapy. A certified medical scanning device is used for all our testing which I am fully qualified and trained to use. Many people like this therapy as they have found it helpful, non-invasive and allows them to feel that they have some control over looking after their own health naturally. However, if you are suffering any serious health condition it is my responsibility to inform you that you must seek medical advice from your GP.

Standard Food Test Template Example

Dear

Thank you for choosing to take a standard food test with Langton Smith Health.

Food sensitivity may be a temporary issue that requires a short period of time to desensitise the body to certain foods. We have found that six weeks to three months is a good period of time to limit the specified foods and allow the body to cleanse itself of those foods that have caused symptoms. These may include bloating, stomach cramps, acidity, IBS etc.

If you are doing this for curiosity then it might help to try eliminating the foods shown in your personal results below.

Helpful Comments

Please remember that not all symptoms are food related.

Some foods may be shown that you do not eat. This is because the medical scanner will identify any potential sensitivity that may occur whether eaten or not.

Understanding your food sensitivity results:

70–100 = **High Priority sensitivity to eliminate or reduce as much as possible**
40–70 = **Medium sensitivity, reduce or limit from diet**
1–40 = **Low Sensitivity, eat sensibly**

Interpreting your results

The results of the test are personal for you and we have found that it is best to leave the foods listed out of your diet as much as possible for at least six weeks to start to see a difference.

Read the *last food listed* along the line after the titles or headings of diet/nutrition. This will be the specific food to watch for. So in the example below, the food to avoid would be Cheddar Cheese rather than all Dairy Products.

Rate
Diet and Nutrition -> Dairy Products -> Cheddar Cheese

Avoid any of the foods listed above that are applicable to your diet for approximately three months so that you can monitor any changes to your health/digestion. As we do not have information regarding your current diet or lifestyle, it might be interesting for you to follow the recommendations above to see if it makes a difference to your overall health.

Symptoms

Please have in mind that this is a *full food test* and not a full health test. This means that food sensitivity may not provide the entire solution to your health symptoms. There may be other types of health tests that we can offer that may be more appropriate to your specific symptoms. It is suggested that you start with the food desensitisation as detailed in your results. Please contact us again if you need to discuss your health symptoms in more detail.

About the test

The standard food test is the most popular of our tests, due to the increase in awareness to reactions to certain foods. It offers 200 food listings in its database and includes many foods and drinks. You will have received the top 30 foods listed from the 200 scanned in the database. Listed below are the food groups tested, but within each group there are many single foods included.

Grains and cereals; dairy products; fats and oils; non-alcoholic drinks; alcohol; herb teas; meat; fish and shellfish; raw fruit; cooked fruit; raw vegetables; cooked vegetables; nuts and seeds; spices; herbs; sweeteners; sugars; metabolism of certain food groups and requested speciality foods.

Our Food Tests are based on bioresonance therapy, a complementary medical approach to health. All tests are conducted using a scanning device which has an EU medical classification and is covered by the European ISO standard regulations. Hair samples are used to identify a variety of health-related issues and each test is tailored to the individual. Whilst there is no quantitative clinical research undertaken in this therapy, there are plenty of testimonials based on its perceived accuracy and effectiveness.

Heading up the team is Julie Langton Smith MSc, bioresonance nutritional practitioner and Naturopath who oversees each food test result letter before it is sent. Our food test service is personalised to each individual and the offer to discuss your test results is made clear so that if there is anything at all that you need clarification on, please do not hesitate to contact us.

Please note that there may be foods listed that you do not like and would not eat but it gives confirmation that these foods are best avoided. If you know that you already have a problem with a specific food type, and have not eaten them for a while, it is quite normal for these foods not to show up as they will not be resonating in the body system.

Not everyone has food sensitivities but these scans show the top foods to watch out for, or a trend for you to avoid certain types of foods.

Please read the guide to food tests attached and always contact us if you are unsure of your results, we are very happy to explain them to you.
Kind regards

Julie Langton Smith
MSc Psych TPACS
Bioresonance Nutritional Practitioner
dip Nutrition and Diet, dip. Bioresonance Therapy Advanced,
dip.Clinical Hypnotherapy dip Anatomy & Physiology & Pathology
Dip Sports and Physical therapy, dip Assessor and Tutor

Guide to Food Tests
Below is some further information about the standard and gold standard full food tests.

Future Food Testing Recommendations
In our experience future food testing is recommended in the following way: people with acute conditions re-test after 3–6 months to monitor changes. Those people with chronic conditions re-test six months to one year and those who are looking for general maintenance and optimising wellbeing re-test each year. This is because the body varies due to lifestyle and other health changes such as hormone imbalances, stress-related issues, sleep deprivation, environmental factors, pollution, electrosmog, pathogens, insect bites and holiday stomach upsets and so on. Please do contact us for further information on this.

Guide to Understanding Your Food Test

High Sensitivity: foods listed with a score of 70–100 represent high sensitivity or extreme dislikes
These foods need to be greatly reduced or ideally completely excluded from your diet for at least six weeks before a difference is noticed by the

body. Sometimes you can reintroduce foods at this time as some foods are those that may have been eaten too regularly or in too much quantity.

Medium Sensitivity: foods listed with a score of 40–70
All foods listed with a score of 40–70 represent medium sensitivity and should be reduced a little from your diet. However, if you eat any of these foods in quantity on a regular basis, then it is recommended that you eliminate these from your diet for a six-week period enabling you to monitor any change to your symptoms.

General Sensitivity
If there is a trend of foods such as grains/wheat etc., which cover numbers across the board, we will include these as a general sensitivity; there will be a recommendation to confirm this if necessary.

What is understood by the terms food allergies, food sensitivities and food intolerances

Allergies
A food allergy is defined by a severe acute reaction to a specific food; this may cause swelling of the tongue, lips and respiratory organs, rapid heart rate, dizziness, skin rash and/or change of skin colour, shaking, upset stomach/sickness or fainting. This can be very frightening and serious. This also means that this food should never be eaten.

Sensitivities
Food sensitivities are mainly defined by the symptoms such as bloating, excessive gas, indigestion, irritable bowel (IBS), loose stools, lethargy, tiredness after eating, skin sensitivities such as dry skin/sore skin, psoriasis, blocked sinuses or excessive mucous and sometimes weight gain. Food sensitivities may cause chronic and long-term health symptoms if not addressed. This indicates that a certain food or food group may need to be avoided for a while before it can be reintroduced to identify whether this is a long-term sensitivity or food intolerance.

Intolerances
The Food Test 400 is designed to help identify food sensitivities. However, if subsequent food tests indicate the same food sensitivities each time it is highly likely that this food becomes a food intolerance which means that it is best left out of the diet long term.

Metabolism
The heading of metabolism means the process of digestion.

Fats suggest that there is a possible problem in processing fats in the digestive system and this can cause acid reflux, indigestion, stomach upset and pain. This means saturated fats such as in cheeses, butter, fatty meats such as beef or lamb, coconut, palm oil, cream and some fish such as sardines. See following link for more information:
http://www.bhf.org.uk/heart-health/prevention/healthy-eating/saturated-fat.aspx (July 12).

Protein Metabolism usually suggests that a more vegetarian type of diet would be suitable for some people.

Acid metabolism suggests that foods either containing acid such as vinegars, pickles or even some fatty foods that convert to fatty acids may also create acidity in the digestive system which then can cause symptoms such as IBS.

A list of Acid / Alkaline Forming Foods

Alkaline Forming Foods

VEGETABLES
Garlic
Asparagus
Fermented Veggies
Watercress
Beets
Broccoli
Brussel sprouts
Cabbage
Carrot
Cauliflower
Celery
Chard
Chlorella
Collard Greens
Cucumber
Eggplant
Kale
Kohlrabi
Lettuce
Mushrooms
Mustard Greens
Dulce
Dandelions
Edible Flowers
Onions
Parsnips (high glycemic)
Peas
Peppers
Pumpkin
Rutabaga
Sea Veggies
Spirulina
Sprouts
Squashes
Alfalfa
Barley Grass
Wheat Grass
Wild Greens

FRUITS
Apple
Apricot
Avocado
Banana (high glycemic)
Cantaloupe
Cherries
Currants
Dates/Figs
Grapes
Grapefruit
Lime
Honeydew Melon
Nectarine
Orange
Lemon
Peach
Pear
Pineapple
All Berries
Tangerine
Tomato
Tropical Fruits
Watermelon

PROTEIN
Eggs (poached)
Whey Protein Powder
Cottage Cheese
Chicken Breast
Yogurt
Almonds
Chestnuts

OTHER
Apple Cider Vinegar
Bee Pollen
Lecithin Granules
Probiotic Cultures
Green Juices
Veggies Juices
Fresh Fruit Juice
Organic Milk (unpasteurized)
Mineral Water
Alkaline Antioxidant Water
Green Tea
Herbal Tea
Dandelion Tea
Ginseng Tea
Banchi Tea
Kombucha

SWEETENERS
Stevia
Ki Sweet

SPICES/SEASONINGS
Cinnamon
Curry
Ginger
Mustard
Chili Pepper
Sea Salt
Miso
Tamari
All Herbs

ORIENTAL VEGETABLES
Maitake
Daikon
Dandelion Root
Shitake
Kombu
Reishi
Nori
Umeboshi

Acid Forming Foods

FATS & OILS
Avocado Oil
Canola Oil
Corn Oil
Hemp Seed Oil
Flax Oil
Lard
Olive Oil
Safflower Oil
Sesame Oil
Sunflower Oil

FRUITS
Cranberries

GRAINS
Rice Cakes
Wheat Cakes
Amaranth
Barley
Buckwheat
Corn
Oats (rolled)
Quinoa
Rice (all)
Rye
Spelt
Kamut Wheat
Hemp Seed Flour

DAIRY

NUTS & BUTTERS
Cashews
Brazil Nuts
Peanuts
Peanut Butter
Pecans
Tahini
Walnuts

ANIMAL PROTEIN
Beef
Carp
Clams
Fish
Lamb
Lobster
Mussels
Oyster
Pork
Rabbit
Salmon
Shrimp
Scallops
Tuna
Turkey
Venison

PASTA (WHITE)
Noodles
Macaroni
Spaghetti

OTHER
Distilled Vinegar
Wheat Corn

DRUGS & CHEMICALS
Aspartame
Chemicals
Drugs, Medicinal
Drugs, Psychedelic
Pesticides
Herbicides

ALCOHOL
Beer
Spirits
Hard Liquor
Wine

BEANS & LEGUMES
Black Beans
Chick Peas
Green Peas
Kidney Beans
Lentils
Lima Beans
Pinto Beans
Red Beans
Soy Beans
Soy Milk
White Beans
Rice Milk
Almond Milk

Nightshade Veggies	Tofu (fermented) Flax Seeds Pumpkin Seeds Tempeh (fermented) Squash Seeds Sunflower Seeds Millet Sprouted Seeds Nuts	Wakame Sea Veggies		Cheese, Cow Cheese, Goat Cheese, Processed Cheese, Sheep Milk Butter	Potatoes	

(http://www.rense.com/1.mpicons/acidalka.htm May 2012).

Sugar/Glucose Regulation often suggests that there is either too much sugar for the body to be able to process adequately or too much in quantity for the body to manage. As each person functions very differently, there will be various amounts that can be absorbed and processed by each person.

Sugars, Carbohydrates and Glucose
Obvious foods that contain sugars are: sweets, sugar, cakes, biscuits, chocolates, honey and molasses.

Sugars are in all carbohydrates and some are considered as fast-releasing sugars such as white starchy foods, for example, potatoes, rice, pasta, pizza or bread, fruit such as melons and grapes and vegetables such as carrots.

When sugars, sugar balance regulation, glucose or carbohydrates appears on the food list it means that a diet low in sugars is preferable. This means that a low glycaemic index (GI) diet should be followed that contains slow-releasing sugars such as brown carbohydrates, rice, pasta and breads. We recommend that fruit such as apples, pears or berries, vegetables such as sweet potatoes and green-leafed veg are eaten regularly.
http://www.the-gi-diet.org/lowgifoods for more information on low GI foods.

Protein Metabolism
We have found that when this is indicated on the test results a more vegetarian style of diet is recommended.

Glycerine
This is found in some medications and sweeteners.

Enzymes
Enzymes are the body's natural chemicals to break down the food we eat. This starts the moment we put food into our mouths and swallow and continues all the way through to complete digestion. Sometimes, at different times in a person's life, perhaps changes in lifestyle, illness, stress, menopause or age, the production of these digestive enzymes changes and the digestion of food becomes slow or creates a sluggish digestion. It may mean that certain foods that used to be eaten become indigestible. When 'enzymes 'appear on the food list it is suggested that perhaps a natural digestive enzyme taken before each meal for a while may help to stimulate the digestion and process of food and may help to ease symptoms.

Raw and Cooked
Sometimes you will see foods mentioned twice and this is due to the difference in the way the body processes raw foods and cooked foods. It is normally understood that if a food is a high value it is best to avoid, whether raw or cooked.

Yeast
Yeasts can show when there is a build-up of fungal activity, which is too much for the body's digestive system to handle. This can result in symptoms such as skin rashes/eczema, bloating, weight gain, tiredness, bladder problems/thrush and general feelings of being under the weather. Always reduce sugars when this is indicated, as well as excluding any foods that contain yeast, such as bread, cakes, buns, beer and so on. Normally taking a good probiotic and not a probiotic yoghurt for six months can help. It might be recommended to have a pathogen and toxin test which may identify what else may be needed.

Ordering Vitamins: Please email us for assistance if you require advice or call.

Professional Disclaimer: Please remember that this is complementary medicine and does not form part of any conventional medical process. I have been practising for many years as a nutritional healthcare practitioner specialising in bioresonance therapy. A certified medical scanning device is used for all our testing which I am fully qualified and trained in using. Many people like this therapy as they have found it helpful, non-invasive and allows them to feel that they have some control over looking after their own health naturally. However, if you are suffering any serious health condition it is my responsibility to inform you that you must seek medical advice from your GP.

Weight Loss Test Template Example

Dear

The results of your personal weight loss food test are listed below. Based on your hair sample these are the top foods that need to be eliminated from your diet; this is not a diet but a personal food plan, by informing you of which foods you personally need to avoid which will help you to lose weight. Remember that there may be other food issues as this is not a full food test but this weight loss food test may give you a good start towards your weight loss goals.

Weight Loss Tips
To achieve best weight loss, food portions needs to be monitored. It is recognised that portions equivalent to the size of a tennis ball are helpful in achieving successful weight reduction. This is because the stomach is designed to digest a specific amount of food at any one time, any more than this results in excess food being converted into fat.

Helpful Comments
Please remember that not all symptoms are food related.

Some foods may be shown that you do not eat. This is because the medical scanner will identify any potential sensitivity that may occur whether eaten or not.

Understanding your Food Sensitivity Results

70-100 = High Priority sensitivity to eliminate or reduce as much as possible
40-70 = Medium sensitivity, reduce or limit from diet
1-40 = Low Sensitivity, eat sensibly

Food Sensitivities and how to start a new diet regime to eliminate foods indicated on my list
These may only be a temporary issue and require a short period of time to desensitise the body to certain foods. We have found that as rule of thumb, three months is a good period of time to allow the body to cleanse itself of foods that have built up and may have created certain health conditions.
Avoid any of these that you eat on a regular basis or eat in quantity and that are applicable to your diet. Try this for at least six weeks and up to

three months so that you can monitor any changes to your health/digestion. We do not have information regarding your current diet or lifestyle so it might be interesting for you to follow the recommendations here to see if it makes a difference to your overall health.

Common Food Sensitivities Explained
Sugars: fast-releasing Carbohydrates

Sugar Cravings are so addictive, more so than salt cravings. Sugars are in so many foods that most of us would not even consider. The other issue to consider is the way in which we cook a food and thereby change its sugar content. Some foods may be fine if boiled but not if they are mashed or roasted and fried. For example, white foods such as rice, potatoes, bread, cakes, pasta, and dairy all contain sugars as they are fast-releasing carbohydrates and therefore convert into sugars. The other sugars that most of us don't realise are the sugars in fruit. The top fruit for high sugar content are most melons, grapes, bananas and pineapple. The lower sugars are in apples, pears and berries such as raspberries and strawberries. Please see the glycaemic index which informs you of the levels of sugars in all foods researched and provided by The University of Sydney. http://www.glycemicindex.com/

Bread: When bread is indicated with a *medium or high* figure, this means it needs to be avoided even if it is wheat or gluten free. This is often due to its consistency, which can be difficult for some people to digest.

Yeast: When yeast is indicated with a *medium or high* figure, this normally means to avoid bread and any food that contains yeast, including foods such as fruit/juices, alcohol (beers, lagers), sweets and refined sugars as these foods act as triggers for yeast growth. It may also be helpful to take a good probiotic capsule for three months to help stabilise the gut flora and support the immune system.

Gluten: When gluten is indicated with a *medium or high* figure, it is recommended to avoid all grains that contain gluten for approximately three months. These include wheat, barley, rye, semolina, spelt and couscous. These are found in foods such as bread (including breadcrumbs), rolls, chapattis, biscuits, crackers, cakes, pastries, pizza, pasta, gravies and sauces etc. Below are examples of some of the foods that contain wheat and gluten.

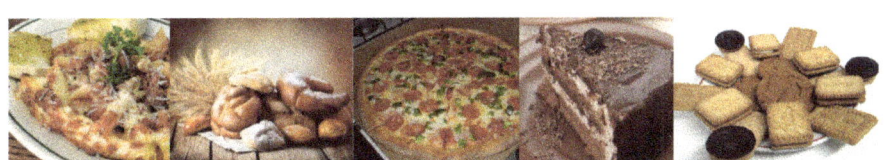

Suggested replacement foods

Corn, rice, rice flour, amaranth, buckwheat, millet, teff, quinoa, sorghum, soya flour, potato starch, modified starch, potato flour, gram flour, polenta (cornmeal), sago, tapioca, cassava.

We do not recommend eating gluten free foods as they tend to be expensive and some are genetically modified to make them gluten free; however, this is your decision to make.

Dairy: When milk is indicated with a *medium or high* figure, it is recommended to avoid *all* dairy. This is because all dairy derives from milk. Below are examples of foods that contain dairy.

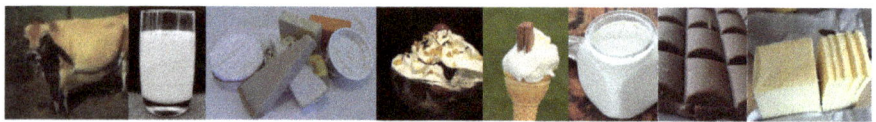

Suggested replacement foods

Dairy-Free
As all dairy originates from a cow, it is advised to adapt your diet to other types of dairy-free or alternatives such as soy, nut milks, rice milks, goat and sheep products.

Feedback – Testimonials
We would be really grateful for any feedback from you, if you have the time, as it is helpful for other people struggling with weight issues and there are many of them. Thank you very much in advance as this is something that we are very serious about and want to know if there has been any improvement in your symptoms.

Symptoms
Please bear in mind that this test is scanning for those foods that you personally need to avoid in order to lose weight and is *not* a full food test. This means that other foods may be sensitive for you and so this test may not provide the entire solution to your health symptoms. We suggest that you start with eliminating the foods listed here, if appropriate for you, and then contact us again if you need to discuss your health symptoms in more detail.

About our other Food Tests
Our food tests are based on bioresonance therapy, a complementary medical approach to health. All tests are conducted using a medical

scanning device which has an EU medical classification and is covered by the European ISO standard regulations (2017). Hair samples are used to identify a variety of health-related issues and each test is tailored to the individual.

Heading up the team is Julie Langton Smith MSc, bioresonance nutritional practitioner and naturopath who oversees each food test result letter before it is sent. All our tests are personalised to each individual and the offer to discuss your test results is made clear so that if there is anything at all that you need clarification on, please do not hesitate to contact us.

Please note that there may be foods listed that you do not like and would not eat, but this test indicates a potential sensitivity that these foods are best avoided. If you know that you already have a problem with a specific food type and have not eaten them for a while it is quite normal for these foods not to show up as they will not be showing a resonance in the body. Always contact us if you are unsure of your results, we are very happy to explain them to you.
Kind regards

Julie Langton Smith MSc
MGHRC, MFHT, MNCS, PSA
Bioresonance Nutritional Practitioner and Psychotherapist

www.langtonsmithhealth.com/

Professional Disclaimer: Please remember that this is complementary medicine and does not form part of any conventional medical process. I have been practising for many years as a nutritional healthcare practitioner specialising in bioresonance therapy. A certified medical scanning device is used for all our testing which I am fully qualified and trained to use. Many people like this therapy as they have found it helpful, non-invasive and allows them to feel that they have some control over looking after their own health naturally. However, if you are suffering any serious health condition it is my responsibility to inform you that you must seek medical advice from your GP.

Chapter 13

Testimonials and Feedback

It is important to receive feedback from patients/clients regarding the service a practitioner offers. The quality of the information is important and whether the results have helped the patient/client with regard to their symptoms.

In this section there are a number of testimonials and feedback emails concerning a variety of health tests, mostly food tests. Anonymity is crucial and therefore the identity of these patients has been kept confidential. These are some of the feedback emails and letters that have been received over the years. Please note that it is important to accept negative feedback even if the overall feedback is good. It is in this way that a good practitioner will modify their work to offer a more comprehensive report for the patient/client.

The practitioner is offering a service to a patient/client that must be customer led. The patient/client is the customer and therefore all feedback is vital for any practitioner to be able to create a successful practice. It is often through receiving some negative feedback that a practitioner can amend the way in which they work to offer a better and more enhanced service.

Keeping ahead of what other practitioners offer is also of great advantage, as knowing what a customer (patient/client) needs from their tests can tailor the work perfectly for a practitioner.

Positive feedback also assists in confirming what the practitioner is doing in the way it has helped the patient/client and in this way can also help other people to see the advantages in having these tests. It is advisable to check that testimonials and feedback can be used in any marketing and advertising in the country that the practitioner is operating in as this can vary.

These are a few samples of the testimonials and feedback, showing a variety of ways of asking patients/clients for some feedback. Whether it is in the form of a questionnaire or an email it makes no difference as long as you take notice of what is said and are grateful to your patient/client for taking the time to do this.

Testimonials:

JC 2017
My sister, my husband and I have all had various tests carried out by Julie Langton Smith and this has helped us massively with our health and digestive issues. Julie is always quick to respond and really helpful with queries that you may have. Just because you have received your test results doesn't mean the service stops there. The post-test service we have received is really impressive and the offer to re-test my iron levels for free to make sure I am back on track is amazing.

We would recommend anyone interested in their health, diet and wellbeing to consider the tests the Langton Smith Clinic has to offer – they are well worth the money.

CM 2017
Dear Julie,
Thank you for your email, and I am very happy to give positive feedback. We went for the standard food allergy test a few months ago, with regard to my 13-year-old daughter suffering from migraines, some of them severe. She has since cut out milk which was one of the main things that you flagged up. She has had only 2 migraines since.

I was pleased with how easy the whole process was, and will be soon doing the food test myself as I suffer from rheumatoid arthritis and am convinced some foods are irritants.
Many thanks, and good luck with the book!
Kind regards

EK 2017
Q & A
Can you list your original symptoms?
Did you follow the test results?
Yes. For the first few months very strictly. Now I allow one meal a week where I can have anything as it's very hard to maintain.

1. What changes did you notice?
   All symptoms went within the first few weeks.

2. How are your symptoms now?
   Triggered when built up in my body. I can have one meal off and I'll be okay. Have mild symptoms but nothing major, but if I was

to have two days in a row the pain is significantly worse.

3. Would you choose this food testing service again?
   Yes without a doubt and I've already told so many people about how it's helped me.

Any other comments

Just that it's a great service you offer and has made my life so much better. Thank you.

KP 2017
I've used Langton Smith twice now for my eldest son and my youngest.

My eldest as an infant had eczema but not severe, however on a night he would itch uncontrollably making for very disturbed sleep. I chose Langton Smith after seeing an offer on Groupon and thought I would give it a go, the best decision I ever made! The results came back showing a high reaction to wheat and a couple of other foodstuffs. We immediately followed the advice and the difference was almost immediate, he stopped itching. If he ever had something with wheat in we could tell as he would start itching again. After about 18 months we reintroduced wheat and he was able to tolerate it with no side effects and now has a full unrestricted diet. Some people told me they didn't believe in how the testing was done and it couldn't be accurate, however, the results speak for themselves!

My youngest was exclusively breast-fed and at just under 12 months we decided to introduce cow's milk as a drink ready to start weaning from me. He had had it in cereal and small amounts but as we upped the quantities he was extremely uncomfortable on a night, writhing in discomfort and would then often comfort feed from me all night which was exhausting, along with explosive nappies. After a holiday in Thailand where he wasn't having much cow's milk we noticed a big difference so I once again turned to Langton Smith. His reaction to cow's milk was 100%, however, other milk products weren't as high so we have kept small amounts of these in his diet. If he has a little too much then you can tell as the explosive nappies come back but he is a lot more settled on a night. We are still following a restricted diet but hopefully soon we can try again, however, I don't think he is ready for more cow's milk yet.

GL 2017
Just to say that I recently had a blood test at my doctor which gave the same gluten result as your test.
Best wishes

AB 2017
I first approached Langton Smith clinic after a period of itching skin, nose bleeds, energy depletion and anxiety. The initial test was the food sensitivity and thereafter a full health test. On both occasions I followed Julie's advice with which foods to eliminate, reduce or avoid plus took the recommended supplements and homeopathic remedies. After the first 3 months the itching skin had stopped and nose bleeds reduced. After the second test and follow-up medicines my nose bleeds have stopped, anxiety levels have significantly reduced and my general energy levels are in balance again.
I can highly recommend the Biofeedback/Bioresonance treatment and support for both mental and physical imbalances. Thank you Langton Smith Clinic for opening up a happier and healthier world for me and my family.

MB 2012
Thank you for sending my results so promptly. I would like to comment on how straightforward the report is, easy to understand and act on. Also thank you for your time in answering some questions I had and knowing I can call again is very much appreciated.

RH 2012
I just wanted to say a big thank you for the results. I was aware of some of the foods on the list which were causing me issues already, such as chocolates, but at the same time there were some which I was surprised about such as tomatoes and lamb. I have noticed that foods which I am sensitive to usually cause me a lot of indigestion and heartburn so hopefully I will now try cutting them out which will hopefully improve the situation.

LC 2012
Thank you for my test results, I started eliminating all the things listed and already in four days I feel better. I just have a couple of
> questions... One of the items said Bread (not a surprise for me) but
> does this include Wraps and Pitta and go as far as including cakes

> etc.? and also two of the vegetables, carrots and peas say (cooked)
> does this mean I can eat these raw ?

LP 2015

Thanks so much for this, I have found it very stimulating reading and was very glad to be able to give some feedback:

FEEDBACK FORM FOR FOOD INTOLERANCE SCAN

We would be very grateful if you would complete this questionnaire and return it to us, so we may know how you felt about your experience with us and improve our service.

	POOR	NEUTRAL	GOOD	EXCELLENT
Was your experience as you expected from a remote scan?				*
Was your scan dealt with promptly and efficiently?				*
If you asked any questions, were these dealt with respectfully?		Didn't ask any questions		
Did you understand the results from your scan clearly?				*
Do you felt it helped you in your day to day life?				*

Do you have any other comments you wish to tell us about?

I actually hadn't really understood the nature of the scan when I bought the Groupon and was a bit sceptical about the whole process. I had thought it was a more 'conventional' kind of test and was not too sure about how all this was supposed to work...

I am a vegetarian who hasn't eaten fish for over 20 years but at the point I was becoming vegetarian became increasingly sure that fish and I did not agree with one another! One of my grandparents was quite strongly allergic to fish so the high reading for that absolutely chimes with the reality of what I already know about myself in one way, but I'm a bit confused as the background information seems to suggest that if you have already eliminated something from your diet it won't be resonating any more? I'd really appreciate a bit of clarification on that if you wouldn't mind please.

I love black olives and was about to put some in a salad for tea until I read this!

I keep toying with the idea of being vegan so I actually don't have much dairy but in the way of using things up – bought for omnivores and not eaten some weeks ago – I have had some cheese the last couple of days and when I took the test had just had pizza – half hot one day, half cold the next – 2 days running at my boyfriend's place! That had mushrooms and black olives added but no feta! It's interesting that the sensitivities are so very specific.
While at his house I also had a white bread (something I never buy!) Marmite sandwich, yeast extract I do like but don't have all that often so will give that a few weeks off too!

I am relieved that wheat didn't show up as I know a number of people that's a problem for and it's a tricky one to completely avoid and I was also glad chilli didn't come up as a friend who loves it turned out to be sensitive to it and I understand that people sometimes love / crave the very things which do them no good!

Reading up on Vitamin A rich foods to remind myself I find that normally these feature quite strongly in my diet but have been entirely absent while I've been away! I usually have a sweet potato with hummus pretty much 5 days a week and as many days probably eat a large carrot and for the time I was away had neither of those things. I have been salad deprived as well – warned off any uncooked veg in Nepal – a real hardship for me!

I'm not really a beer fan but had a bit a couple of times on holiday in the first few days and thought I didn't dislike it as much as I thought but didn't really fancy having it again so didn't! Avoiding it will be no hardship! Yeast also an issue there.

I never normally drink Coke but while I was away had it a couple of times as a bit of an antidote to stomach upset as it's supposed to contain the right balance of salt and sugar to rehydrate, but since coming home have had no intention of drinking it again, so easily avoidable too.

Interestingly I can't think when I last had Ovaltine but a Horlicks is not unknown, I guess if Horlicks had been a problem – or malt extract which I sometimes have in milk rather than buying Horlicks, that would have shown?

I am very fond of bean soups and had to Google to remind myself what English people call Lima beans and was relieved to see butter beans don't feature in the Tuscan bean soup I've had the last few days and the pumpkin soup I had earlier today will boost the vitamin A count too.

So I have found this all very interesting.

FEEDBACK FORM FOR FOOD INTOLERANCE SCAN

We would be very grateful if you would complete this questionnaire and return it to us, so we may know how you felt about your experience with us and improve our service.

	POOR	NEUTRAL	GOOD	EXCELLENT
Was your experience as you expected from a remote scan?				√
Was your scan dealt with promptly and efficiently?				√
If you asked any questions, were these dealt with respectfully?				√
Did you understand the results from your scan clearly?				√

Do you felt it helped you in your day to day life?				√

Do you have any other comments you wish to tell us about?

The results have been very interesting! When I rang up to discuss them, all my questions were answered clearly and concisely. The therapist (not sure if that is the correct term, sorry!) that I spoke with was very helpful and polite.

Thank you very much.

Thank you for your time in completing this.

Chapter 14

How to Become a Successful Practitioner

Professional Guidelines for Working as a Bioresonance/Biofeedback Practitioner

It is always vital to consider the business of working as a practitioner, understanding what is needed to work in this field of therapy, the codes of practice, the regulations and the laws. Please always check with your own country's laws and regulations so that you are covered in offering 'best practice' for your client/patient. Below are some examples and information for any practitioner to consider as part of their working practice.

Code of Ethics including Confidentiality, Disclaimers and Professional Insurance to Practice

Code of Ethics
The code of ethics describes the basic ethical principles that all the complementary health practitioners agree to and commit themselves to.

The practitioner must hold full professional indemnity insurance. Insurance is to be maintained at all times and must be recognised in the country where the practitioner is and cover all aspects of the health modalities practised.

All patient/client information records must be kept absolutely confidential and secure at all times.

For supervision, research, teaching and publication purposes, the identity of the patient/client must be concealed.

The practitioner must be able to determine whether a patient/client requires conventional medical attention in the case of serious illness. In this case it is the practitioner's responsibility to encourage the patient/client to seek advice from their GP. The practitioner will need to ensure that they have noted all information in their case history notes and if necessary ask the patient to sign that they have been advised to seek medical advice by the practitioner. This then ensures the practitioner has upheld the professionalism and also may assist if any serious situation arises.

Patients/clients under the age of eighteen will need parents/guardians written consent for any health check or test.

The practitioner will only undertake a formal therapeutic relationship with the patient/client whilst treatment is underway. Any other relationship/friendship and such like can only commence once the therapeutic/patient/practitioner relationship has ended.

The patient's/client's beliefs must be respected at all times.

The patient's/client's dignity and integrity must be respected at all times.

Adverts in all forms must abide by the British Code of Advertising Practice. Practitioners may not advertise or promote themselves in any other way than what they are qualified to do. They must not use the words, 'cure' or attempt to give the impression that they are able to offer any remedy unless they are qualified to do so.

The practitioner and patient/client agree a clear contract which addresses precisely and openly the questions of fees, time involved, frequency and number of sessions, technique of treatment, limits and ground rules, confidentiality, availability of follow-up and referrals. This ensures full disclosure and assists in setting the ground rules for the relationship and treatment between the practitioner and the patient/client.

Hygiene is of high importance and must be upheld at all times. Premises must be of a good professional standard. All equipment must be kept in a hygienic condition.

The practitioner must inform their patients/clients of any change in circumstances such as a move of premises or retirement. It is important that the practitioner make provisions for the continuance of their care. In the event of the practitioner's death, preparations should also be made so that clients are notified.

Practitioners should not speak disrespectfully of other therapists in public, to clients or to students. Respect other practitioners and health professionals.

Practitioners are responsible for continuing their professional development (CPD) through training, supervision and study.

In the case of any complaint, this should be first addressed directly to the practitioner and/or then to their professional association.

Do not mislead your clients or make any false claims of your skills and abilities.

Disclaimers

Example:
Disclaimers are important for all practitioners as it helps to clarify the extent of the area of treatment or therapy being given to a patient/client. This means that if there is a serious illness or condition, the patient/client can see from the beginning the limits of a practitioner's expertise. It is entirely up to the practitioner how they wish to communicate their limits and extents of treatment for a patient/client but it is strongly advised that this is conducted in writing from the very beginning so that there is no room for confusion.

Disclaimers are important on all marketing literature, websites and letters to patients/clients. They help to protect the practitioner and the patient from unreal expectations for cures, remedies and treatment and also helps to keep all therapies offered by the practitioner strictly in accordance with their qualifications, training and insurance cover. Here is an example of a couple of disclaimers but do check with the country you are working in to ensure that you have covered all aspects of a disclaimer for your specific type of work.

Example of author's disclaimer:
Professional Disclaimer: Please remember that this is complementary medicine and does not form part of any conventional medical process. Julie Langton-Smith has been practising for many years as a nutritional healthcare practitioner specialising in bioresonance therapy that is based on a medical scanning device that Julie is fully qualified and trained in using. Many people like this therapy as they have found it helpful, non-invasive and allows them to feel that they have some control over looking after their own health naturally. However, if you are unsure of your health in any way or suffering any serious health condition it is recommended that you seek medical advice from your GP.

A guide to a general disclaimer which covers all aspects of marketing including websites:

Disclaimer: If you require advice relating to a serious condition or illness, it is strongly advised that you contact your doctor or other medical practitioner.

You should never delay seeking medical advice, disregard medical advice, or discontinue medical treatment because of information on this website.

Name of practitioner or health company are not qualified to provide advice about serious health problems and nothing in the content of this website constitutes any form of medical advice. Any natural complementary health care information provided is not to replace any conventional medical attention that the patient may require.

Name of practitioner or health company specifically disclaims all responsibility for any liability, loss or risk, personal or otherwise, which is incurred as a consequence, directly or indirectly, of the use and application of any of the information on this site.

Professional Insurance
The complementary and alternative practitioner/therapist will need to ensure that they have adequate insurance. This will need to include public liability insurance which covers the practitioner in case a person is injured or their property is damaged due to your business in anyway. If there are contractors, people employed employers liability insurance will be needed even if you are working from home you will need this insurance. You may also require business premises insurance, so it is always best to check to make sure you are covered for everything you need. Ensure that all the types of therapies practiced are listed on your policy form or you will not be covered. If you work with children ensure that you have the appropriate paperwork and insurance to do this. There are a number of insurance companies that specialise in CAM therapies in the UK and Internationally.

Data Protection

Example:
What is GDPR?
The General Data Protection Regulation (GDPR) will be enforced across Europe, including the UK. The law aims to give citizens more control over their data and to create a uniformity of rules to enforce across the continent.

Coverage Scope
The GDPR covers all data controllers and data subjects based in the EU. It also applies to organisations based outside the EU that process the personal data of its residents.

According to the EC, the definition of personal data covers anything that points to their professional or personal life, including names, photos, emails, IDs, bank details, social networking posts, medical information, or computer IP address.

There will be a Single Data Protection Authority (DPA) assigned to each company depending on where the company is located who will report to the European Data Protection Board. They must be appointed for all public authorities and companies processing more than 5000 data subjects within 12 months.
(sourced 12/2/18 https://www.getfilecloud.com/blog/2015/02/a-dummys-guide-to-eu-data-protection-laws/#.WoGkJkx2vid**)**

The rules can be seen as following 6 themes:
1. Know what you have, and why you have it
2. Manage data in a structured way
3. Know who is responsible for it
4. Encrypt what you wouldn't want to be disclosed
5. Design a security aware culture
6. Be prepared

(Source 12/2/18, https://nilehq.com/journal/gdpr-for-dummies/**)**

Proof of Consent
Data controllers must possess a valid proof of consent for processing data and acquire special permissions for collecting the data of children under 13 from their legal guardians.
Data will be collected, stored and used in a manner that ensures it is relevant, timely, accurate, coherent, transparent and accessible.

Please ensure that you are aware of the most up-to-date laws and regulations so you are fully insured to practise.

Chapter 15

Conclusion

The final part of this book sums up all the work here and tries to explain objectively the reasons of working with energy and the importance of the bioresonance practitioner's training, knowledge and experience in this process.

The chart below indicates the results from a patient's point of view (interviews carried out independently), and may help to show how this all comes together to form a very safe, effective and progressive therapy for future medicine.

It wouldn't be true to say that there are no question marks over any complementary and alternative medical therapy and it is with a scepticism that I entered into this area of CAM. Informed criticism is useful. In other words those who are accusatory of any CAM therapy need to have a better understanding of said therapy before they become negative and critical. However, it is fair to say that we all have a different way of thinking about life, some people are very logical and streamlined in their approach to problem solving and others are very creative and lateral in their approach. I believe a bit of both is necessary to have a level head and even with no clinical evidence, as yet, the anecdotal evidence based on qualitative research is significant. If a person receives positive benefit from any CAM therapy it needs to be accepted and respected.

One of the issues with bioresonance and biofeedback therapy is the way in which the results are not easily replicated as not all tests appear to show the same results on two subsequent scans, immediately one after the other. Energy never remains the same; it is always shifting, which is why results may vary. This may appear to be too random but to an experienced practitioner they will be able to interpret the results by assimilating the results and identifying the priorities that have been indicated on both scans. However, this can be confusing to both patient and practitioner. Only by practising with these devices and understanding them, will the practitioner feel confident in understanding the results. This is why training is vital as many 'lay' practitioners are not experienced enough or trained to a level of competence to ensure 'best practice'. Using the biofeedback/bioresonance devices in the correct way and by programming in the symptoms correctly before doing the test will help the practitioner to receive the best results. However, it is vital that the practitioner knows how to interpret the results by correlating them with the symptoms presented. If the practitioner is not knowledgeable enough, there runs a risk that the symptoms and the foods listed from the test may not make sense to the patient. There is anecdotal evidence available to help validate this work; no clinical trials have been conducted and as in most CAM therapies, the therapy results would not be measurable in a clinical trial as yet. Nevertheless, qualitative research has been carried out.

The positive aspects of working as a bioresonance practitioner is the ease with which the device can be used. This includes the use of non-invasive methods such as hair samples and no clinic visits are necessary, thus making this therapy more accessible to those patients/clients who cannot travel and even practitioners who are unable to travel for whatever reason. Results from tests have helped many of the patients who have given testimonials and in this section there is further information concerning the effect of having had bioresonance and biofeedback therapy. Whilst some of the points raised are varied between the therapist/practitioner's personal energy and the therapy itself, I would argue that this is one and the same. No complementary therapy can be practised unless the practitioner/therapist is at one with the therapy. This flow of energy from practitioner and the bioresonance/biofeedback device will help to provide the patient with the best results; the practitioner will then be able to interpret the results more accurately for the patient. This interpretation is based on the results from the device, but dependant on the practitioner's knowledge and experience and ability to explain their meaning in accordance with the list of symptoms the patient has presented. The ease with which the assessment is done and the information provided has proven to help thousands of patients over the years. Whilst qualitative research has been carried out and therefore based on anecdotal evidence this can be argued as a strong point too as the experience of individual patients feeling the benefit from having bioresonance and biofeedback therapy has been clearly stated in this research.

Research Results
This final section is a snapshot of the research carried out and attempts to sum up the perceived effectiveness of bioresonance and biofeedback therapy from the patient's point of view.

Ten participants were interviewed independently; they had all had full health tests and a range of symptoms. The participants were a mix of male and female and all ages. Names have been changed to protect their identities.

There were common goals among the respondents and these represented the main themes. The goal attainment scale was used to explore what the respondents' goals were at the beginning of therapy and whether these had been achieved. They were asked to rate these according to their experience in numbers from -2 = very unsuccessful through to +2 = very successful. The table below identified these 3 main themes by these respondents.

Goal Attainment Findings

Personal Goal Attainment	Mary	Edith	Peter	Laura	Mike	Susan	Anne	Gwen	Paula	Kath
Wanting to know what the problem was – confirm or affirm	+2	+2	+2	+2	+2			+2	+2	
What to do about it – solutions	+2	+2	+2	+2	+2	+2	+2	+2	+2	+2
Overall wellbeing and advice for future healthcare	+2	+2	+2	+2		+2	+2	+2		+2

All participants were seeking to understand what their health problem was, confirm what they may have thought; just to find out what was wrong and all wanted to find solutions. These were best described in the part of the discussion interview when the respondents were asked what their goals were when they entered the therapy.

This study was based on a sample of ten participants who have expressed their views based on their personal experiences.

There were four big themes that emerged and have been outlined as main topics for further discussion. The sample demonstrates the background of the participants and their profiles, what they entered the therapy with, including their ages, personal information such as health issues and employment history; there is a range of people who seek CAM therapies even on this small sample. It would be interesting to study further into demographic profiles of people who choose a CAM therapy (Chua & Furnham, 2008). It also emerged that all those who sought CAM therapies in this study were originally attracted to doing so because they had a health problem that had not been successfully diagnosed or treated in a way that they were satisfied with through their own GP. This demonstrated a vulnerability when entering a CAM therapy as they were unwell, dissatisfied with conventional treatment, looking for more answers and therefore more likely to be open to trying other methods of approaching their health and wellbeing.

The choice of bioresonance therapy appears to be either based on personal recommendation through a member of the family/friend or having read an article about the therapy.

The majority of participants presented attitudes that were 'open minded' in seeking help through CAM therapies. Motivating factors for choosing and using CAM therapies included prevention, wanting to know what the problem was, a holistic approach that embraced the body and mind (Hyland, Lewith and Westoby, 2003) as well as the emotional body, spending more time discussing their health, a tailor-made and personalised approach to their health and wellbeing, finding solutions that included natural ways of healing such as foods to avoid and nutritional therapy. Whilst some of the participants mentioned their disillusionment with their GP and conventional medicine, they all claimed to understand that the GPs are under pressure and have no time to give them a tailored personal and holistic approach (Heiligers, de Groot, Koster and van Dulmen ,2010).

All participants claimed that their health goals on entering this therapy had been fulfilled. Words used to describe the therapy included: it works, felt hopeful, saw change straight away, found solutions, feel better, reassuring and pinpointed problems.

Although the reasons for choosing CAM therapies are many as described, it can be prohibitive for some due to the expense. Most of the participants have used bioresonance therapy on an annual or bi-annual basis for monitoring changes in the wellbeing of their body. This can become expensive and is therefore a reason for this therapy to run the risk of becoming elitist in that only those who can afford it will continue for the long term or that people will drop out due to its cost (Chua & Furnham, 2008). It could be argued that due to the fact that there is a charge for CAM therapies, this could raise the expectations of the patients in feeling that they are paying for something to feel better.

Explaining the hair sample for repeat scans did appear to be a credibility issue for some of these respondents and may be an area that needs further thought, although it did not stop these participants from pursuing follow up scans. It may be an issue for its use in future medicine.

When these participants approach the therapy they suspend any belief even to the point of not wanting to know how it works. Most described it as being connected to the hair or magnetics, frequencies and energy, yet none of them actually said that it was a priority for them to know. This could be further argued in conventional medicine as to how many people know how instruments such as MRI and X-ray machines actually work. All respondents in this sample acknowledged that it was important to follow the instructions given to them from the Bio Scan and that their healing process would improve the more compliant they were. The relationship with the therapist was important and the word 'trust' and/or 'faith' was used by many in the sample (Verhoef, Lewith, Ritenbaugh, Boon, Fleishman, Leis, 2005). The ability to communicate and feel that there is both a professional and friendly rapport was also apparent for the majority. Anchoring their belief was supported by BRT 'picking up on things' that the participants could relate to without having already said anything previously, connecting physical symptoms to stress-related mind/emotional problems and vice versa and reinforcement of things that were already known by the participant and not disclosed, as already mentioned in the perceived effectiveness section.

The subject of bioresonance and its place in future medicine included issues such as its perceived ability to detect and assess certain health symptoms in this sample, things that had not been disclosed but the patient knew about prior to BRT. Furthermore, it is argued that there was evidence from this sample that conventional medical testing, such as blood tests and X-rays, carried out after the bioresonance scans had discovered specific health symptoms and then validated its findings. Most of this sample believed that the perceived success was a combination of therapist and therapy, although the argument for using the bioresonance instrument on its own purely as a diagnostic tool was a major finding. There were many in this sample who would like to see this therapy used as a diagnostic tool in GPs' surgeries and this would therefore further emphasise that the bioresonance tool itself may have a place in future medicine.

About the Author

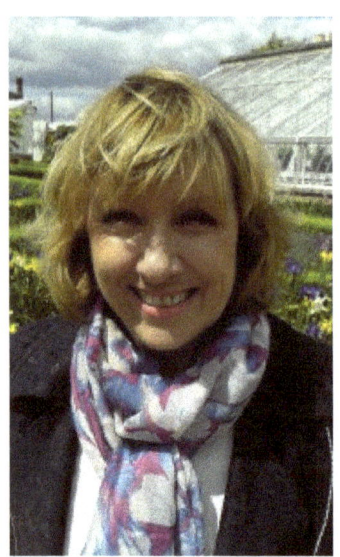

Julie Langton Smith MSc

Julie is a naturopathic specialist who combines psychology, psychotherapy, coaching and clinical hypnotherapy as an overall approach to assessing the health of each individual. She has more than twenty years' experience of working in natural health.

Julie's approach to her treatments as a naturopath involve biofeedback and bioresonance therapy (digital health assessment) using a certified biofeedback scanning device that offers test results for food intolerances, digestive system issues, vitamin deficiencies and full health testing using hair samples.

The powerful connection between the mind and body provides a unique approach to the overall health of each individual therefore Julie wanted to further validate her work by doing a Master's Degree in Transpersonal Psychology and Consciousness Studies at the University of Northampton. This allows for a more mindful, spiritual and human approach to health issues bringing in a deeper understanding of some of the underlying reasons for symptoms ranging from weakened immunity, IBS, weight fluctuations, headaches, insomnia, cravings, back and joint pain. Having qualified as a psychotherapist, she offers a choice of treatments with the aim of looking at both the physical symptoms and the mind/emotion connection involved in the symptomatology presented. Combining NLP coaching, psychotherapy/counselling and clinical hypnotherapy she is able to offer help with a range of issues ranging from anxiety, panic, phobias, bereavement including pet bereavement, addictions, family and relationship counselling, psychosomatic blocks to help with fertility, menopause and hormone balance, skin conditions and coaching for life and business changes.

She has also worked in HMP Lewes (Her Majesty's Prison) as a counsellor and coach to help the rehabilitation of men back into everyday life.

Having worked in Horsham, West Sussex, UK for twenty years, and Harley Street, London for seven years, she is now in Littlehampton, West

Sussex, UK and has set up a private consulting room for clinical hypnotherapy, psychotherapy/counselling for individuals, group and business therapy sessions. She heads the team for food, vitamin and general health testing using certified digital medical scanning equipment.

Background and Qualifications: Julie's career started in healthcare in the late 1980s with a little known therapy at the time called neuro linguistic programming. She continued her studies in anatomy, physiology and pathology (function, structure and pathology of the human body), advanced training in sports physio and physical therapies (physio at the Horsham Rugby club), then progressing on to complementary therapies such as kinesiology and nutrition and diet, bio magnetic therapy, homeopathy and acupuncture.

Dip. Anatomy, Physiology and Pathology, dip. Nutrition and Diet, dip. Sports and Electrotherapy, D32/33 Assessor City and Guilds, dip. Kinesiology, dip. Bioresonance Therapy (Advanced), dip. Advanced Clinical Hypnotherapy and Past Life Regression, dip. Psychotherapy and Counselling, MSc Psychology (Transpersonal and Consciousness Mindfulness Studies). Research Paper on the 'Perceived Effects of Bioresonance Therapy', University of Northampton, UK.

Lectures and Articles and Training: Julie is an experienced practitioner who has lectured at the University of Westminster, London, Association for Fibromyalgia and the Association for Systematic Kinesiology. She has been featured in Health Sections of *Spirit & Destiny*, *Best Magazine*, *Body Language*, BBC and author of *Slim Now with Fish*, a booklet sponsored by Nestlé and what was known as The White Fish Authority in the '80s. Julie has also lectured in anatomy/physiology and pathology as well as nutrition and diet, offering accredited diplomas in these subjects.

Author of nine audio titles – 'Hypnotherapy for Health', which are available as downloads. These offer specific sessions in a range of health subjects for Insomnia, (Sleep Talk Lullaby with Des'ree), You Tube views have reached more than 500,000. Other titles include Menopause, IBS, Anxiety, Terminal illness, Behavioral Issues, Smoking, Weight Loss and Heart Disease.

Acknowledgements and Contributions

A huge thank you to Emma who worked very hard on the nutritional chapter in this book and has been a great support in the world of bioresonance.

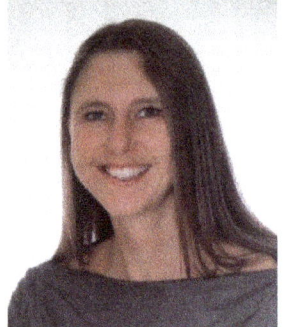

Emma has worked in bioresonance therapy for over ten years. She has always been interested in alternative health and throughout her career as a dance teacher has been fully aware of the powerful impact nutrition has on the body. With this keen interest, Emma completed qualifications in both anatomy and physiology and diet and nutrition and is now a nutritional adviser and bioresonance/biofeedback practitioner.

Emma Sewell: dip. Nutrition and Diet (distinction) dip. Anatomy Physiology and Pathology. dip fstbt food testing consultant

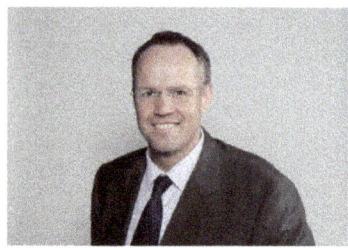

Also a massive thank you to Harald Rauer who has been kind enough to write the chapter on the principles of how bioresonance and biofeedback therapy is perceived to work. This has been invaluable information.

Harald Rauer MSc

Studied Information and Systems Engineering (MSc.) in Munich.
Since 1989 he has researched Subtle Energies and Information Medicine, Radionics and Reichs Orgonomy.
Studies of 'Radionics' and 'Psychotronics' in USA.
Former president of the German Radionic Association (DRG e. v.)
Member of the British Radionic Association.

In 1997 he joined a research team to develop the first, automatic computer-aided testing devices.

As a result of this cooperation he developed the computer-aided Resonance System MARS III, implementing for the first time a completely new technology based on 'Tesla coils', which has never been used in this field before.

As a result of the research going into the MARS III, he left the principles of 'Radionics' behind, and worked towards a conversion to a scientifically

based 'Quantum Response Technology'®, which incorporates the base of Energy and Quantum medicine.
Shareholder and Managing Director of Bruce Copen Laboratories.

References:

Adams, J (2007) *Researching Complementary and Alternative Medicine*

Ali, M. (2001) *Integrated Health Bible*

Barlow, F & Lewith, G. (2009) *The ethics of complementary therapy research recruitment. British Journal of General Practice,* April 2009, 302–303

Brugemann, H (2006) "are there evidence-based studies on the efficacy of bioresonance therapy?", Int.Med.Association BICOM Bioresonance Therapy (IMABRT) paper given during the International Medical Association Congress held April 2006 in Fulda

Chua,S & Furnham, A (2008) *Attitudes and beliefs towards complementary and alternative medicine (CAM): A cross-cultural approach comparing Singapore and the United Kingdom Complementary Therapies in Medicine* (2008) 16, pages 247–253

Copen, B (1999) A *Materia Medica of Homeopathic Formulas*

Dawson, C. (2007), *A Practical Guide to Research Methods*

Dawson, C (2009) Introduction to research Methods

Foucault, M. (1972) *Power/Knowledge*

Geller, U. (1999) *Mind Medicine*

Gerber, R. (2000) *Vibrational Medicine for the 21st Century*

Glaser, B. and Strauss, A. (1999) *Discovery of Grounded Theory: Strategies for Qualitative Research*

Grafman, J. (2009) *National Institute of Neurological Disorders & Stroke*, March 2009

Greenfield, T (1996) Research Methods, guidance for post graduates

Heiligers, P.,[1,2] Judith de Groot,[1,3] Dick Koster,[4] and Sandra van Dulmen
[1]*Diagnoses and visit length in complementary and mainstream medicine,* BMC Complement Altern Med. 2010; 10: 3.
Published online 2010 January 25. doi: 10.1186/1472-6882-10-3.

Heistand, D. & S., (2001) *Electrical Nutrition*

Hollway, W & Jefferson, T (2000) *doing qualitative research differently*

Howarth, D, (2000) *Discourse*

Hyland, M. Lewith, G & Westoby (2003) *Developing a measure of attitudes: the holistic complementary and alternative medicine questionnaire, Complementary Therapies in Medicine, Volume 11, Issue 1,* March 2003, Pages 33-38

Lewith, G, Jonas, B & Walach, H (2002) *Clinical Research in complementary therapies*

Marshall, P. (1997) *Research Methods, How to design and conduct a successful project*

Oldfield, H. & Coghill, R. (1988) *The Dark Side of the Brain*

Peters, D. (2005) *Family Guide to Complementary and Conventional Medicine,* Page 14

Potter, J., Wetherell, M., 1995, *Discourse analysis*

Reyner, J. Laurence, G. & Upton, C. (2001) *Psionic Medicine*

Sheldrake, R. (1999) *Dogs that know when their owners are coming home*

Schneider, R & Walach, H.,(2006) *Randomized Double-Blind Pilot Study on Psychological Effects of a Treatment with 'Instrumental Biocommunication'* Institute for Environmental Medicine and Hospital Epidemiology and Samueli Institute Europe, University Hospital, Freiburg, Germany (Forsch Komplementarmed 2006)

Smith, J., Flower, P., Larkin, M., (2009) *Interpretative Phenomenological Analysis, Theory, Method, research*

Smith, JA(2008) Interpretative phenomenological analysis. In JA Smith (ed) *Qualitative Psychology: A Practical Guide to Methods.* London: Sage Willig, C. (2001). *Introducing qualitative research in psychology. Adventures in theory and method.* Buckingham: Open University Press. (Chapter 4)

Smith, J.A., Jarman, M., & Osborn, M. (1999). Doing interpretative phenomenological analysis. In M. Murray & K. Chamberlain (Eds.), *Qualitative*

Snow, D.A. & R.D. Benford. 1988. *Ideology, Frame Resonance and Participant Mobilization*

Solomon, J & Solomon, G. (1998) *Harry Oldfield's Invisible Universe*

Strauss, A & Corbin, J, (1997) *Grounded Theory in Practice*

Thomas, K & Coleman, P,(2004)*Journal of Public Health* Vol. 26, No. 2, pp. 152–157, DOI: 10.1093/pubmed/fdh139 Printed in Great Britain

Website References:
http://www.parliament.uk/documents/commons/lib/research/rp99/rp99-111.pdf (Hicks, J., Allen, G, 1999) House of Commons **RESEARCH PAPER 99/111 (**21 DECEMBER 1999) retrieved 4.6.2010
www.radionic.co.uk/what_is_radionics.htm retrieved May 09

http://www.energetic-medicine.net/search/search.php?zoom_query=white+noise retrieved June 2010

http://www.copen.com/indexMAIN.php?sprache=English&parent=22&child=0 (Bruce Copen Labs retrieved June 2010)

http://www.geos.ed.ac.uk/geography/Ethics/form1.html retrieved

 11th Feb 2010

http://www.ico.gov.uk/upload/documents/library/data_protection/practical_application/the_guide_to_data_protection.pdf

retrieved 11th Feb 2010

http://www.radionic.co.uk/ retrieved 9th December 2009

http://www.legislation.org.uk/ retrieved 16th December 2009

Rothstein.G, Trends in Mortality in the 20th Century,1995

Lee. Philip, Estes. Carroll, The Nations Health, 2007

http://www.dcp2.org/pubs/DCP/1/Section/114 - June 2009
http://www.parliament.uk/commons/lib/research/rp99/rp99-111.pdf - June 2009

U.S. Dept of Health and Human Services
http://nccam.nih.gov/news/camstats/2007/camsurvey_fs1.htm
http://www.dh.gov.uk/en/Publicationsandstatistics/Publications/PublicationsStatistics/DH_4006687
Developing Patient Partnerships
http://www.dpp.org.uk.
http://www.askaboutmedicines.org .
Medical News Today
http://www.medicalnewstoday.com/articles/17554.php
Foundation for Integrated Medicine
www.fih.org.uk

Web Refs May 17
http://aetherforce.com/a-very-brief-history-of-radionics-by-ruth-drown/
http://www.radionics.org/09_radionics_history_1.html
http://aplaceforhealingvm.com/radionics/
http://quwave.com/Scalar-Waves.html

http://www.healingintowellness.co.uk/scio-quantum-biofeedback-therapy/
https://bioresonance.com/therapy-machine/

July 17
Read more at https://www.penguin.co.uk/books/1025042/psionic-medicine/#ZuG2U18gCbXViCEj.99
http://www.nicko500.co.uk/MGA.htm

https://www.google.co.uk/url?sa=i&rct=j&q=&esrc=s&source=images&cd=&cad=rja&uact=8&ved=0ahUKEwjjs87ukPnTAhXL1RoKHRBTBhwQjhwIBQ&url=http%3A%2F%2Fwww.keywordsuggests.com%2Fhuman-digestive-system-diagram-showing%2F&psig=AFQjCNH7sTF-g9DxN2B-PmWeM0Mxu9rdtA&ust=1495186165489001

Bioresonance Accredited training courses available please see website http://www.bioresonancetraining.com

Our courses are led by Julie Langton Smith MSc and are available to UK and international English speaking students. All our courses specialise in the therapy of bioresonance/biofeedback. Bioresonance/biofeedback courses require a bioresonance device. Please contact info@bioresonancetraining.com for further information.

Accredited Bioresonance Practitioners Worldwide

Sweden and UK

Annalisa Börjesson

Langton Smith Health

Nutritional Consultant & Food Sensitivity Practitioner

Passionate for happy, healthy, organic living.

http://langtonsmithhealth.com/blog/

UK

Emma Sewell

Intolerance Testing For You

http://www.intolerancetestingforyou.com

Email: evsewell@hotmail.com

Nutritional adviser and bioresonance/biofeedback practitioner and have worked in the area of Biofeedback and Bioresonance therapy for over 10 years. Offering food intolerance and vitamin and mineral testing.

Australia

Anna Talaj ND

ATNatural Therapies

naturopath@atnaturaltherapies.com.au

GUT health specialist, Naturopath and Nutritionist who is passionate about helping you achieve your optimal health.

Spain

Philippa Harvey MSc

http://www.harveyhealth.net

info@harveyhealth.net

Integrative practitioner with over 15 years' experience in complementary healthcare

TCM practitioner, MPEFTOS, Practitioner number 10702-867, MSc Applied Psychology, BA.hons Business Management

www.ingramcontent.com/pod-product-compliance
Lightning Source LLC
Chambersburg PA
CBHW040521220526
45473CB00013B/2935